Scholarly Inquiry
and the DNP Capstone

Cheryl Holly, EdD, RN, ANEF, is professor and chair, Department of Capacity Building Systems, co-director of the Northeast Institute of Evidence Synthesis and Translation at Rutgers School of Nursing, and a fellow in the Academy of Nursing Education. She teaches doctor of nursing practice (DNP) program courses, including information technology for evidence-based practice, systematic review, and meta-analysis, and works with DNP students in their capstone residency course. Dr. Holly holds a Bachelor of Science in Nursing from Pace University, Leinhard School of Nursing, Pleasantville, New York, where she was named a distinguished alumna; a Master's in Education in adult health and physical illness; and a Doctor of Education in research and evaluation in curriculum/teaching, both from Columbia University. In addition, Dr. Holly has completed postgraduate work in financial administration at the New York Medical College School of Public Health and studied economics and accounting at Pace University School of Business. She has also taken postgraduate courses in comprehensive meta-analysis. Among many other positions held, Dr. Holly previously was director of nursing research and informatics at New York University Langone Medical Center in New York City; senior vice president of quality clinical resource management at the Westchester Medical Center; and associate dean, Columbia University School of Nursing. She is certified as Train-the-Trainer in comprehensive systematic review by the Joanna Briggs Institute and has offered workshops on comprehensive systematic review across the country. Dr. Holly is the coordinator of the Eastern Nursing Research Society's Research Interest Group on Comprehensive Systematic Review and Knowledge Translation, and a member of the Committee on Directors of the Joanna Briggs Institute of Nursing and Midwifery, the Evidence Translation Group, Cochrane Nursing Care Field, the Cochrane Injuries Group, and the Joanna Briggs Institute Methodology Group on Umbrella Reviews. She serves as manuscript reviewer for several journals, including *Nursing Outlook, Nursing Education Perspectives, American Journal of Nursing,* and the *Journal of Critical Care Nursing.* Dr. Holly has been principal investigator, co-principal investigator, or project director of eight funded research projects. She has published extensively and presented internationally and nationally in the areas of evidence-based practice, systematic review, knowledge translation, and critical care nursing.

Scholarly Inquiry
and the DNP Capstone

Cheryl Holly, EdD, RN, ANEF

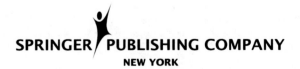

SPRINGER PUBLISHING COMPANY
NEW YORK

Springer Publishing Company, LLC
11 West 42nd Street
New York, NY 10036
www.springerpub.com

Acquisitions Editor: Margaret Zuccarini
Composition: S4Carlisle Publishing Services

ISBN: 978-0-8261-9387-2
e-book ISBN: 978-0-8261-9388-9

13 14 15 16 17 / 5 4 3 2 1

The author and the publisher of this Work have made every effort to use sources believed to be reliable to provide information that is accurate and compatible with the standards generally accepted at the time of publication. The author and publisher shall not be liable for any special, consequential, or exemplary damages resulting, in whole or in part, from the readers' use of, or reliance on, the information contained in this book. The publisher has no responsibility for the persistence or accuracy of URLs for external or third-party Internet websites referred to in this publication and does not guarantee that any content on such websites is, or will remain, accurate or appropriate.

Library of Congress Cataloging-in-Publication Data
Scholarly inquiry and the DNP capstone/[edited by] Cheryl Holly.
    p. ; cm.
Includes bibliographical references and index.
ISBN-13: 978-0-8261-9387-2
ISBN-10: 0-8261-9387-0
ISBN-13: 978-0-8261-9388-9 (e-book)
I. Holly, Cheryl, editor of compilation.
[DNLM: 1. Clinical Nursing Research—methods. 2. Advanced Practice Nursing.
3. Research Design. WY 20.5]
RT81.5
610.73072–dc23
                                    2013036020

Printed in the United States of America by Gasch Printing.

As with all things I do, this book is dedicated to Bebe, Grace, and the guys.

CONTENTS

Angelito S. Antonio, DNP, APN
Nurse Practitioner
UnitedHealthcare
Flemington, New Jersey

Donna Barto, DNP, RN, CCRN
Advanced Nurse Clinician
Virtua Health
Marlton, New Jersey

Mary Jo Bugel, PhD, RN, CNL, CNE
Assistant Professor and Director of Graduate Adjunct
   Faculty Development
Coordinator, MSN in Clinical Leadership
Rutgers School of Nursing
Newark, New Jersey

Keesha A. Duncan, DNP, APN, CCRN
Co-Chief Anesthetist
Jersey City Medical Center
Jersey City, New Jersey

Mercedes Echevarria, DNP, APN
Assistant Professor
Assistant Dean, DNP Program
Rutgers School of Nursing
Newark, New Jersey

Rosario P. Estrada, DNP, RN, BC, CPN
Assistant Professor/Track Coordinator
Nursing Informatics MSN Program
Rutgers School of Nursing
Newark, New Jersey

Maryanne M. Giuliante, DNP, GNP, ANP-C
Nurse Practitioner
Memorial Sloan-Kettering Cancer Center
New York, New York

Joan Harvey, DNP, RN, CCRN
Nurse Educator
Ocean Medical Center–Meridian Health
Brick, New Jersey

Deneen Scuderi, MSN, RN
Director of Nursing Education
Westchester Medical Center
Valhalla, New York

Jackeline Biddle Shuler, DNP, JD, RN
Attorney and Health Care Consultant
Long Branch, New Jersey

Ahmad Singer, DNP, PhD, RN, FACHE
Associate Executive Director
Emergency Department
Perioperative Services
Cancer Center
Queens Hospital Center
Queens, New York

REVIEWERS

Mercedes Echevarria, DNP, APN
Assistant Professor
Assistant Dean, DNP Program
Rutgers School of Nursing
Newark, New Jersey

Rosario P. Estrada, DNP, RN, BC, CPN
Assistant Professor/Track Coordinator
Nursing Informatics MSN Progam
Rutgers School of Nursing
Newark, New Jersey

Marybeth Lyons, MSN, RN
Clinical Nurse Specialist
Pediatrics and Pediatric Intensive Care
Westchester Medical Center
Valhalla, New York

Lisa M. Paplanus, DNP, ACNP-BC, ANP-BC, RN-C, CCRN
NP Coordinator, Vascular/General/Bariatric Surgery
NYU Langone Medical Center
New York, New York

A scholar is a learned person—someone who has studied for a long time and gained mastery in a discipline. By nature, advanced practice nurses are practice scholars, having studied a long time to gain the expertise and knowledge necessary to provide safe and cost-effective patient care across a variety of practice settings. As experts in a practice discipline, nurses think critically about the problems they face and question what they are doing. This book is intended to support that inquiry, not through the development and testing of theory, but rather through practice-based studies. The intended audiences are advanced practice nurses, students in advanced practice nursing programs, and doctoral students interested in conducting clinically based studies. Faculty may also benefit from this book. The content selected reflects my work with doctor of nursing practice students over an 8-year period.

The book is presented in two parts. The first part is about scholarship. Chapter 1 describes the nature of nursing practice. Being a scholar and engaging in scholarly inquiry require an understanding of the nature of practice and what it means to be a scholar. The value of understanding the complex relationships among practice, clinical wisdom, and reflection is that knowledge grows from practice, and it is practice that provides an avenue for a scholarly practice, and therefore, inquiry. Chapter 2 introduces the concept of scholarly inquiry developed around the four domains of Boyer's model of scholarship: application, discovery, integration, and teaching.

The second part addresses the methods of scholarly inquiry that lend themselves to clinical investigation. Chapter 3 introduces action research, a reflective process about research in action. Action research is grounded in context, and involves real-world situations and problems. It is a constantly evolving method of inquiry conducted within familiar settings by teams working together for the resolution of practice problems. Chapter 4 describes case study research. Constructing a case study is an opportunity to highlight success, to bring attention to a particular challenge or difficulty, or to describe a unique or unusual event. The case study method allows investigation of a clinical problem within a particular context bounded by time, place, and activity, and in which multiple sources of evidence are used. Chapter 5 is about qualitative descriptive research. This method is used when a direct description of events using the terms provided by the subject is sought. It is the preferred method when an uncomplicated description is desired. Chapter 6 is about clinical interventional research. Because nursing is a practice discipline, an understanding of how particular interventions work and in what context they work can inform practice and improve patient care. Chapter 7 discusses systematic review. A systematic review is a descriptive research method in which the subjects or informants in the study are published or unpublished primary studies, rather than human subjects. Systematic reviews are an accepted form of research, the findings of which are used by practitioners to make point-of-care decisions based on the best available evidence for a focused clinical question. Chapter 8 is about integrative review, a critical summary of literature on a particular topic. An integrative review appraises and combines available evidence, including theory. It takes a traditional review of the literature one step further by providing a more substantial contribution to knowledge using a transparent process, and making a critical appraisal of the literature used in the review. New perspectives and frameworks can be generated through an integrative review, and research questions can be developed. Chapter 9 is on quality improvement. The focus of quality-improvement activities is on systems and processes that can be improved. The last chapter, Chapter 10, is on program evaluation. A program evaluation is the process of collecting, analyzing, and using data to measure the impact or outcomes of a program. Typically, evaluation involves assessment of one of the following: (a) program need, (b) program plan, (c) program performance, (d) program impact, or (e) program effectiveness.

My aim is to provide a useful resource to those who desire to engage in clinical research projects. To supplement this information, I asked several of my former doctoral students and colleagues to develop an expanded abstract of their doctoral project. Examples of each of the methods contained in this book can be found following each chapter.

Advanced practice nurses have the ability to develop clinically focused practice projects that cannot only advance nursing practice, but also inform the redesign of health care in light of new and emerging health care mandates, and inform primary research.

Cheryl Holly

ACKNOWLEDGMENTS

I wish to express my sincere thanks to all of my doctor of nursing practice (DNP) students, past and future, who have helped shape the project designs presented in this book. The work involved in a DNP capstone project is intense and sometimes difficult. It is also immensely important and directly related to safe, quality patient care. I am motivated and encouraged every time I read about the outcomes of their projects. My special thanks and gratitude to all of you.

I also wish to thank Dr. Mary Jo Bugel and Ms. Deneen Scuderi, who, while not my students, were gracious in allowing me to use their fine work as an example of action research.

This book would not have been possible without the support and guidance of Margaret Zuccarini of Springer Publishing Company, who was extremely patient with me as I missed deadline after deadline.

I

Scholarship

Being a Scholar

OBJECTIVES

At the end of this chapter, you will be able to:
- Explain the nature of professional practice
- Describe strategies to support interprofessional collaboration
- Develop a plan for scholarly practice

KEY CONCEPTS

- Practice is an intentional activity shaped by experience and meaning.
- Experienced practitioners have the capacity to adapt to the complex phenomenological aspects of practice.
- A wise clinical nurse is able to make choices and take action without knowing in advance quite what the consequences will be.
- A reflective practitioner is one who both learns from experience and about experience.
- Inherent in being wise is the understanding that interprofessional collaboration is necessary for optimal patient outcomes.

Being a scholar and engaging in scholarly inquiry require an understanding of the nature of practice. Although scientific practices predominate in most settings, there are contextual issues that differ. According to Pearson (2011), "Expert nurses possess deep sensitivity to the social, cultural and biological contexts of their patients and an ability to adapt rapidly to the unpredictable day-to-day dynamics of the hospital, clinic or community" (p. 443). In other words, the nature of nursing practice is more than the concepts propagated by curricula and standards. It is essential for clinical nursing scholars to keep this in mind as they inquire into the nature of nursing practice. A practice is personal, based on experiences, and experienced practitioners have the capacity to adapt to the complex phenomenological aspects of practice. Intuition may play a role in this adaptation as Schraeder and Fischer (1986, p. 161) have commented, "intuitive perception in nursing practice is the ability to experience the elements of a clinical situation as a whole, to solve a problem or reach a decision with limited concrete information." In other words, there is a "gut feeling" or sixth sense at play without benefit of analysis (Rew & Barrow, 1987). According to Ruth-Sahd (2003), intuition is a key element in discovery, holistic problem-solving, understanding, and knowledge generation. Dossey, Keegan, and Guzzetta (2003) identify six characteristics of nursing intuition:

- Pattern recognition—the ability to put things together given disparate pieces
- Similarity recognition—the ability to see resemblances and compare them
- Common sense and understanding
- Skilled know-how
- A sense of salience—knowing what is right and most important
- Deliberate rationality—the ability to think about things with a purpose in mind

Rew and Barrow (1987) concluded in a study of nurses' intuition that nurses reflect on the meaning and consequences of acting on limited information, which both mitigates the linear approach of the medical model and enhances nursing practice. This chapter focuses on the nature of nursing practice in a real-world context, a discussion in which clinical wisdom and reflective practice contribute, and where intuition, knowing, and skill are overarching components.

CHARACTERISTICS OF PRACTICE

According to Gilgun (2010), "practice takes place in particular situations at particular times with particular persons within a complex set of contingencies that affect practitioners, service users, their interpretations and meanings, and how they engage with each other" (p. 10). In other words, individuals are embedded in events, attribute meaning to each of these events, and, based on these meanings, they practice.

Kemmis (2006) tells us that practice is not just an activity; rather, it involves intentional action and draws on disciplinary knowledge, personal knowledge, and technical knowledge. According to Kemmis (2006), practice is shaped by experience, is culturally located, employs learned competencies, and is frequently regulated through law or policy. Practice involves practical and critical reasoning about how to act in given situations, which allows development of a professional role. Carper's four fundamental ways of knowing have been used as a framework for practitioner development (Carper, 1978). The four patterns are: empirical knowing, esthetic knowing, ethical knowing, and personal knowledge (Table 1.1). According to Carper, "there is a need to examine the kinds of knowing that provide the discipline with its particular perspectives and significance. Understanding four fundamental patterns of knowing makes possible an increased awareness of the complexity and diversity of nursing knowledge" (p. 21). Understanding the complex interplay among these four patterns allows exploration of the various concepts linked to nursing's educational, evaluative, and practice processes (Zander, 2007). In illustration, Zander (2007) relates this story from her time working

TABLE 1.1   Nurses' Ways of Knowing

Way or Pattern of Knowing	Foundation	Characteristics	Example of a Question for Inquiry
Empirical	Science Theories Models Principles	Objective Verifiable	What is the effect of noise on blood pressure?
Esthetic	Art Skill Experience	Intangible Individual	What is the meaning of advanced nursing practice to those who practice it?
Ethical	Morality Philosophy Personal values	Rights Duty	What moral principles are evident in nurses' decisions regarding end-of-life care?
Personal	Authenticity	Awareness of self Interpersonal relationships Engagement	How do nurses describe their role in patient situations where the patient lacks autonomy?

Source: Carper (1978); Zander (2007).

in the Marshall Islands with a group of nursing students from the United States:

> A Marshallese man from one of the outer islands had been brought to the hospital for an emergency below the knee amputation of his right leg. He was septic and for the first few days existed on intravenous (IV) fluids. After his condition improved from very critical to critical, he demanded that the IV be removed. The patient's doctor ordered Gatorade to replace the fluids and electrolytes formerly provided by the IV. The patient refused to drink it. Upon informing the author of their patient's refusal to drink the Gatorade, the students were instructed to ask the man's wife to give him some water from the coconuts she had in the room *(esthetics)*. The students were shocked and asked for rationale for this direction. During a prior experience in the Marshall Islands the author had been told about coconut water being used during the Second World War when no IV fluids were available *(empirics)*. After this episode, a special relationship or bond developed between the Marshallese man, who wanted to be in charge of his situation, and the author, who he allowed to take charge when necessary *(personal)*. (p. 10)

These patterns are also seen in several studies on the characteristics of professional nursing practice. Girard, Linton, and Besner (2005), for example, found that collaboration was the most prominent characteristic of practice, and that professional nursing practice means "working in partnership with other nurses and health professionals in providing client care, being highly organized in managing activities and time, having the ability to manage many complex tasks simultaneously, working autonomously as appropriate and having an open mind and nonjudgmental manner" (para. 9). Competence and commitment were also seen as important components of a professional practice model. A professional practice evolves, according to Riley and Beal (2013). To practice professionally requires constant learning. In a qualitative study of the meaning of scholarly practice, Riley and Beal (2013) found that practice development followed a pattern of recognition that this was a journey from being timid and unknowing to recognizing personal learning needs in situations in which the nurse realized she needed greater knowledge and experience. Finally came the appreciation that patients assisted in practice development. The need to answer patient and family questions requires the nurse to simplify complex information for both her own and the patient's learning. Riley and Beal explained that although nurses were emphatic in their belief that patients saw them as caregivers, not learners, they saw themselves as learners on a journey toward being knowledgeable, comfortable, confident, and skilled practitioners.

CLINICAL WISDOM

Being wise implies that one is shrewd, intelligent, astute, and clever. Confucius (551–479 BCE) wrote, "By three methods we may learn wisdom: first, by reflection, which is noble; second, by imitation, which is easiest; and third by experience, which is the most bitter." Clinical wisdom is about knowledge, experience, empathy, integrity, resourcefulness, and inspiration. Benner, Hooper-Kyriakidis, and Stannard (2011) posited that clinical wisdom is based on clinical judgment and a thinking-in-action approach that encompasses feelings, emotions, and senses with the acceptance that there is an intellectual process and knowledge base made visible through actions and deeds (Haggerty & Grace, 2008). The distinctive features of wisdom include recognition of contextual factors and the place of each person in a situation (McKie et al., 2012). In other words, clinically wise nurses have the ability to connect theoretical physiological signs with patient presentation, and find or develop the resources necessary to ensure optimal patient outcome. They are able to respond quickly and appropriately to patient events. According to Seiden (2010), clinically wise nurses act on behalf of patients who are unable to act for themselves, prevent crises, and assume clinical leadership as needed. The wise nurse who achieves wisdom is tolerant of diversity and differences.

In a study of Danish nurses, Uhrenfeldt and Hall (2007) found that clinically wise nurses made decisions based on changes in patients' conditions. Assessing situations was connected to the nurses' thinking and ethical discernment, transparency about actions taken, and setting of mutual goals with patients. Calmness, assessment of situations, and focusing on patient responses all were essential to decision making. The researchers noted that the barrier of unhealthy working conditions may lead the wise nurse back to nonproficient performance, threatening the nurse's ability to think and act with responsibility.

Inherent in being wise is the understanding that collaboration is necessary. Collaboration is a process of cooperation and teamwork-centered mutual goals. The act of collaborating is usually considered a necessary component of success among individuals or departments within a given organization or between organizations, as well as with patients and families. D'Amour and Oandasan (2005) delineated the concept of interprofessionality as part of the background work for initiatives by Health Canada as:

> the process by which professionals reflect on and develop ways of practicing that provides an integrated and cohesive answer to the needs of the client/family/population. . . . [I]t involves continuous interaction and knowledge sharing between professionals, organized to solve or explore a variety of education and care issues all while seeking to optimize the patient's participation. . . . Interprofessionality requires a paradigm shift, since interprofessional practice has unique characteristics in terms of values, codes of conduct, and ways of working. These characteristics must be elucidated. (p. 9)

Collaboration implies working together for the greater good, but it actually encompasses far more. Collaboration involves teams working on mutually developed and shared objectives. Communication must be straightforward and courteous, keeping in mind the overall intent of the objectives of the team's work. Although collaboration has been associated with teamwork, there is more to successful collaboration. Effective collaboration across health care situations requires explicit, appropriate tasks and goals; clear, meaningful roles for each individual; and clear leadership and feedback on performance (Reeves & Lewin, 2004). In an ethnographic study, Reeves and Lewin (2004) investigated interprofessional collaboration in a hospital setting. They found that the organization itself was composed of individual and isolated nursing units and that the task-oriented nature of hospital work limited opportunities for collaboration with other professionals. Consequently, collaboration tended to be task based, time limited, and formal. The lack of time, staff turnover, lack of knowledge, lack of commitment to the process, and failure to attend meetings emerged as themes in this study.

Effective interprofessional collaboration requires that team members share common perceptions and expectations of each other's roles. A systematic review of five studies on the effectiveness of interprofessional collaboration found that daily discussion or rounds showed a positive impact on length of stay and total charges, and that monthly multidisciplinary team meetings improved prescribing of psychotropic drugs in nursing homes (Zwarenstein, Goldman, & Reeves, 2009). Although beyond the scope of this chapter, an expert panel representing disciplines of nursing, medicine, pharmacy, dentistry, and public health have developed a set of core competencies for interprofessional collaborative practice. The domains include: value and ethics related to interprofessional practice, role and responsibilities of collaborative members, effective communication strategies, and the nature of teams and teamwork (www.aacn.nche.edu/education-resources/ipecreport.pdf). See Table 1.2 for examples of interprofessional collaboration in action.

REFLECTION

Being clinically wise implies an honesty to one's self gained through an examination of one's own practice through reflection. Reflection is an "imaginative, creative, nonlinear, human act" designed to recapture an experience and evaluate it (Ruth-Sahd, 2003, p. 488). Reflective practice allows new discoveries based in the practice situation to emerge (Durgahee, 1997, p. 211). Dewey (1933) first introduced the idea of reflective practice, stating that "reflective thinking is closely related to critical thinking; it is the turning over of a subject in the mind and giving it serious and consecutive consideration" (p. 3). He noted that those who are reflective are open minded and responsive to their experiences. According to Denner (2009), reflection causes a change in brain activity,

TABLE 1.2 Literature-Based Examples of Interprofessional Collaboration

Goldman, J. (2010). Interprofessional collaboration in family health teams. An Ontario-based study. *Canadian Family Physician, 56*(10), e368–e374.

McAlister, F. A., Stewart, S., Ferrua, S., & McMurray, J. J. (2004). Multidisciplinary strategies for the management of heart failure patients at high risk for admission. *Journal of the American College of Cardiology, 44,* 810–819.

Naughton, B., Mylotte, J., Ramadan, F., Karuza, J., & Priore, R. (2001). Antibiotic use, hospital admissions, and mortality before and after implementing guidelines for nursing home-acquired pneumonia. *Journal of the American Geriatrics Society, 49,* 1020–1024.

Phelan, A., Barlow, C., & Iversen, S. (2006). Occasioning learning in the workplace: The case of interprofessional peer collaboration. *Journal of Interprofessional Care, 20*(4), 415–424.

Wang, T., & Bhakta, H. (2013). A new model for interprofessional collaboration at a student-run free clinic. *Journal of Interprofressional Care, 27*(4), 339–340. doi:10.3109/13561820.2012.761598

Zwarenstein, M., & Bryant, W. (2000). Interventions to promote collaboration between nurses and doctors. *Cochrane Database of Systematic Reviews,* (2), CD000072.

specifically increases in alpha and theta waves. This increase occurs particularly in the right hemisphere of the brain, which is associated with insight and "the sudden awareness of correct answers" (Denner, 2009, p. 326).

Professional practice, according to Schon (1983, 1990), is unique and complex. To practice in a professional manner requires reflection as a means of learning from experience. He makes a distinction among three methods of reflection: reflection-in-action, reflection-on-action, and reflection-for-action. Reflection-in-action is a spontaneous reflection in the middle of the action, essentially, "thinking on your feet" (p. 26). It is a conscious, spontaneous action that may be difficult to describe when asked. Reflection-on-action is about thoroughly reviewing a situation after it has occurred; for example, conducting a root cause analysis following an adverse event. In this way, alternative methods of action can be determined should the situation occur again. Reflection-for-action allows a practitioner to determine how further action will be guided. Schon believed that individual practitioners choose their own theories on which to act, rather than blindly accepting what they were taught. He stated:

> In the varied topography of professional practice, there is a high, hard ground which overlooks a swamp. On the high ground, manageable problems lend themselves to solution through the use of research-based theory and technique. In the swampy lowlands, problems are messy and confusing and incapable of technical solution. The irony of this situation is that the problems of the high ground tend to be relatively unimportant to individuals or to society at large, however great their technical interest may be, while in the swamp lie the problems of greatest human concern. (Schon, 1992, p. 54)

DEVELOPING A SCHOLARLY PRACTICE

The value of understanding the complex relationships among practice, knowing, clinical wisdom, and reflection is that knowledge grows from practice; an active practice provides the foundation for scholarly practice and, therefore, inquiry. Perhaps the single most important point in developing a scholarly practice is the desire to want to discover something new and then share it (Hauptman, 2005). Communities of practice, which are groups of people with a common interest and a shared passion who interact regularly, can assist in developing practice-related scholarship (Wenger, 2004). The community is built around shared knowledge, rather than a task. Active engagement by community members is essential. Learning arises out of the act of social participation and evolves through collaboration over time (Andrew, Tolson, & Ferguson, 2008).

Geographic separation is not an issue, as those with shared goals in scholarship can develop or enhance a scholarly practice through the use of technology. By using technology, communities of practice can bring groups together to share expertise and enhance scholarship. For example, a community of occupational therapists met virtually to discuss cases, integrate evidence with experience, identify gaps, shape practice, and improve outcomes. Focused on community mental health, this group comprises Canadian occupational therapists who work together to integrate a model of recovery into their practice (White, Basiletti, Carswell, & Head, 2008). The outcome of their effort was a model of best practice that is now used across Canada. Nurses, collaborating both in real time and online, formed a community of practice to address outdated practices and to promote professional development in the area of gerontology (Tolson, McAloon, Hotchkiss, & Schofield, 2005). The community developed and tested best practice statements (www .geronurse.com).

CONCLUSION

Being a scholar and engaging in scholarly inquiry require an understanding of the nature of practice, a willingness to be involved in new situations, reflection on current practice, confidence, and commitment (Riley & Beal, 2013). Dyck (2012) outlined 10 steps in developing a scholarly practice:

1. Knowing what scholarly activity is about is an important first step. Research is only a part of scholarly activity. To begin requires reflection on the situations around us. To put it metaphorically: A man is walking down the beach and he sees a rock. He pauses and thinks, "I wonder what's under that rock?" He starts to dig and discovers a fish skeleton. The man sees another fellow walking down the beach and yells: "Hey! Want to see what's under this rock?" (p. 1043)

2. Be prepared to find areas for scholarship in any situation.

3. Work on something you're passionate about.

4. Turn a project into a study.

5. Find and heed a voice of wisdom.

6. Learn the basics of Excel.

7. A statistician (or librarian) is your friend.

8. Achieving statistical significance for the first time is cause for celebration.

9. Writing one page (or one paragraph or one sentence) a day for the final report keeps the stress away.

10. Scholarly activity begets new scholarly opportunities.

REFLECTIVE EXERCISES

1. Think about a new practice situation you experienced recently. To reflect on your experience, complete these sentences:
   - "I felt . . ."
   - "I was most anxious about . . ."
   - "I expected my colleagues to . . ."
   - "I learned . . . "
   - "Next time, I will . . ."
   - "I would like to inquire about . . ."
2. Spend a few minutes thinking about your last year in school. What were your goals then? What were your priorities? Have your priorities changed since then?
3. Develop a plan for development of your scholarship over the next 5 years. What do you hope to accomplish, what are your goals, and how will you achieve these goals?

REFERENCES

Andrew, N., Tolson, D., & Ferguson, D. (2008). Building on Wegner: Communities of practice in nursing. *Nurse Education Today, 28,* 246–252.

Benner, P., Hooper-Kyriakidis, P., & Stannard, D. (2011). *Clinical wisdom and interventions in critical care* (2nd ed.). Philadelphia, PA: Saunders.

Carper, B. A. (1978). Fundamental patterns of knowing in nursing. *Advances in Nursing Science, 1*(1), 13–23.

D'Amour, D., & Oandasan, I. (2005). Interprofessionality as the field of interprofessional practice and interprofessional education: An emerging concept. *Journal of Interprofessional Care, 19*(Suppl. 1), 8–20.

Denner, S. S. (2009). The science of energy therapies and contemplative practice. A conceptual review and application of zero balancing. *Holistic Nursing Practice, 23*(6), 315–334.

Dewey, J. (1933). *How we think: A restatement of the relation of reflective thinking to the educative process* (2nd ed.). New York, NY: Heath & Company.

Dossey, B. M., Keegan, L., & Guzzetta, C. E. (2003). *Holistic nursing: A handbook for practice.* Boston, MA: Jones & Bartlett.

Durgahee, T. (1997). Reflective practice: Decoding ethical knowledge. *Nursing Ethics, 4*(3), 211–219.

Dyck, C. (2012). The scholarly path. *Canadian Family Physician, 58*(9), 1042–1043.

Gilgun, J. (2010). *The nature of practice in evidence-based practice.* Paper presented at the Theory Construction and Research Methodology Pre-Conference Workshop, National Council on Family Relations, Minneapolis, MN. Retrieved from http://www.scribd.com/doc/38917585/The-Nature-of-Practice-in-Evidence-Based-Practice

Girard, F., Linton, N., & Besner, J. (2005). Professional practice in nursing: A framework. *Nursing Leadership, 18*(2). Retrieved from www.longwoods.com/content/19028

Hagarety, L., & Grace, P. (2008). Clinical wisdom, the essential foundation of good nursing care. *Journal of Professional Nursing, 24,* 235–240.

Hauptman, R. (2005). How to be a successful scholar: Publish efficiently. *Journal of Scholarly Publishing, 36*(2), 115–119.

Kemmis, S. (2006). What is professional practice. In K. Clive (Ed.), *Elaborating professional practice.* London, England: Springer. Retrieved from http://www.csu.edu.au/research/ripple/docs/Kemmis%20Prof%20Practice%20Chapter%2020060419_14.pdf

McKie, A., Baguley, F., Guthrie, C., Jackson, C., Kirkpatrick, P., Laing, A., . . . Wimpenny, P. (2012). Exploring clinical wisdom in nursing education. *Nursing Ethics, 19*(2), 252–267.

Pearson, A. (2011). Nursing science and practical wisdom: The pillars of nursing knowledge. *International Journal of Nursing Practice, 17,* 443.

Reeves, S., & Lewin, S. (2004). Interprofessional collaboration in the hospital: Strategies and meanings. *Journal of Health Services Research & Policy, 9*(4), 218–225.

Rew, L., & Barrow, E. (1987). Intuition: A neglected hallmark of nursing knowledge. *Advances in Nursing Science, 10*(1), 49–62.

Riley, J. M., & Beal, J. A. (2013). Scholarly nursing practice from the perspectives of early-career nurses. *Nursing Outlook, 61*(2), e16–e24.

Ruth-Sahd, L. (2003). Reflective practice: A critical analysis of data-based studies and implications for nursing education. *Journal of Nursing Education, 42*(11), 488–497.

Schön, D. (1983). *The reflective practitioner: How professionals think in action.* London, UK: Basic Books.

Schön, D. A. (1990). *Educating the reflective practitioner.* San Francisco, CA: Jossey-Bass.

Schön, D. A. (1992). The crisis of professional edge and the pursuit of an epistemology. *Journal of Interprofessional Care, 6,* 49–63.

Schraeder, B., & Fischer, D. (1986). Using intuitive knowledge to make clinical decisions. *Journal of Maternal-Child Nursing, 11,* 161–162.

Seiden, H. M. (2010, Summer). The wild and the wise: Searching for clinical wisdom. *Psychologist-Psychoanalyst,* pp. 19–20.

Tolson, D., McAloon, M., Hotchkiss, R., & Schofield, I. (2005). Progressing evidence-based practice: An effective nursing model? *Journal of Advanced Nursing, 50*(2), 124–133.

Uhrenfeldt, L., & Hall, E. (2007). Clinical wisdom among proficient nurses. *Nursing Ethics, 14*(3), 387–398.

Wenger, E. (2004). Knowledge management as a doughnut: Shaping your knowledge strategy through communities of practice. *Ivey Business Journal, 68*(3), 1.

White, C. M., Basiletti, M. C., Carswell, A., & Head, B. J. (2008). Online communities of practice: Enhancing scholarly practice using web-based technology. *Occupational Therapy Now, 10,* 6–7.

Zander, P. (2007). Ways of knowing in nursing: The historical evolution of a concept. *Journal of Theory Construction and Testing, 11*(1), 6–11.

Zwarenstein, M., Goldman, J., & Reeves, S. (2009). Interprofessional collaboration: Effects of practice-based interventions on professional practice and healthcare outcomes. *Cochrane Database of Systematic Reviews, 3,* CD000072.

SUGGESTED READING

Carper, B. A. (1978). Fundamental patterns of knowing in nursing. *Advances in Nursing Science, 1*(1), 13–23.

D'Amour, D., & Oandasan, I. (2005). Interprofessionality as the field of interprofessional practice and interprofessional education: An emerging concept. *Journal of Interprofessional Care, 19*(Suppl. 1), 8–20.

Dyck, C. (2012). The scholarly path. *Canadian Family Physician, 58*(9), 1042–1043.

Kitson, A. (2006). From scholarship to action and innovation. *Journal of Advanced Nursing, 55*(5), 543–545.

Rolfe, G. (2005). The deconstructing angel: Nursing reflection and evidence based practice. *Nursing Inquiry, 12*(2), 78–86.

Wilson-Barnetta, J., Barriballb, K. L., Reynolds, H., Jowett, S., & Ryrie, I. (2000). Recognising advancing nursing practice: Evidence from two observational studies. *International Journal of Nursing Studies, 37,* 389–400.

The Process of Scholarly Inquiry

OBJECTIVES

At the end of this chapter, you will be able to:
- Explain Boyer's model of scholarship
- Explain the components of a research proposal

KEY CONCEPTS

- Scholarship in nursing concerns those activities that advance the profession.
- All scholarly inquiry starts with a question that guides the entire project.
- Developing a plan to conduct the study is an iterative process.

Scholarship in nursing involves activities that advance the profession through teaching, research, and practice (American Association of Colleges of Nursing [AACN], 1999). According to Boyer (1990), scholarship is generally thought to be related to research; however, the work of a real scholar involves "stepping back . . . looking for connections, building bridges between theory and practice, and communicating one's work" (p. 16); in other words, reflecting. Boyer outlined four domains of scholarship: application, discovery, integration, and teaching. Inquiry into any one of these domains can provide support for evidence-based practices, and each has a specific delineation of what comprises scholarly inquiry. See Table 2.1 for examples in each area of scholarship.

The *scholarship of discovery* is about investigation and the "advancement of knowledge" (Boyer, 1990, p. 17). The scholarship of discovery takes the form of primary empirical research and a variety of qualitative and quantitative methodologies are used, including experimental,

TABLE 2.1 Types of Scholarship

Scholarship Focus	Definition	Examples
Discovery	Generating new knowledge	Publishing in peer-reviewed journals
		Data-based presentations
		Producing creative work
		Research grants
		Research awards
Integration	Synthesizing knowledge for use	Conducting systematic reviews
		Writing a textbook
		Writing book chapters
Application	Addressing problems using knowledge	Serving as a consultant
		Assuming leadership roles in professional organizations
		Advising/mentoring student leaders to foster their professional growth
		Publication of case studies
		Quality-improvement studies
		Operational or program grants
		Peer evaluation
		Specialty certification
Teaching	Achieving optimal learning	Mentoring or precepting students
		Evaluating programs
		Developing instructional materials
		Advancing learning theory through classroom inquiry
		Developing and testing instructional materials
		Mentoring doctoral-student projects
		Mentoring new faculty
		Designing and implementing a program-level assessment system
		Assessment of student learning needs/styles
		Curriculum revision based on current trends and evidence
		Teaching awards
		Development of accreditation reports

Adapted from AACN (1999).

quasi-experimental, descriptive, exploratory, case studies, and ethnography, as well as theory development and philosophical inquiry. The scholar asks, "What needs to be known?" and sets about to find the answer.

The *scholarship of integration* is about synthesis, giving meaning to isolated facts, and putting them in perspective. In other words, illuminating data in different ways, making connections across disciplines, and seeking to interpret findings and generate new patterns for practice. The scholar asks: "What do the findings mean?" Such analysis can lead the scholar from information to knowledge, and "perhaps even wisdom" (Boyer, 1990, p. 19).

The *scholarship of application* is about relevance and service. This element of scholarship is the most practical in that it seeks out ways in which knowledge can solve problems and serve the community, including the professional community. To be considered scholarly service, activities need to flow from professional activity, where theory and practice interact. "Practice scholarship encompasses all aspects of the delivery of nursing service where evidence of direct impact in solving health care problems or in defining the health problems of a community is presented. Competence in practice is the method by which knowledge in the profession is both advanced and applied" (AACN, 1999, para. 18). The scholar asks: "How can knowledge be applied to problems, and how can I help?"

The *scholarship of teaching* is the central element of all scholarship. This element recognizes the daunting work that goes into mastery of knowledge as well as the presentation of information so that others might understand it. "Teaching, at its best, means not only transmitting knowledge, but transforming and extending it as well—and by interacting with students in creative ways" (Boyer, 1990, p. 21). In this context, students also include patients. The construction of a knowledge base comprised of methods, approaches, and activities designed to help assist learning, remembering, and applying subject matter is a primary focus. The identification of methods, approaches, activities, and devices faculty members use to help students understand difficult concepts for specific content or activities constitutes another important aspect of the construction of this knowledge base. Investigation into the effectiveness of untested approaches can be conducted. "The scholarship of teaching is conducted through application of knowledge of the discipline or specialty area in the teaching-learning process, the development of innovative teaching and evaluation methods, program development, learning outcome evaluation, and professional role modeling" (AACN, 1999, para. 15). The scholar asks: "What works best to help my students (patients) learn?"

If works of scholarship in any of these domains are to be accepted, they need to be characterized by a clearly focused clinical question, a clear understanding of research in the field, use of appropriate methods, and reflective critique of the process.

A FOCUSED CLINICAL QUESTION

The decisive activity in any investigation is asking the right question. According to Kitchenham (2004), the right question is one that:

- Is consequential and important to both practitioners and researchers
- Will lead to changes in practice or validation of current practice
- Addresses commonly held beliefs and reality

Developing a research question starts with reflecting on a broad area of concern. Consider, for example, this very general question:

Is obesity a health problem in America?

This is a very broad question, although it provides a focus (obesity and health) and a population (Americans). Proceeding from this point requires that the key components for the study be delineated according to the PICO format. These key components are:

- Patient/population
- Intervention
- Comparison
- Outcome

When describing the *population* it is important to describe the population of primary interest and the important characteristics of the population that are salient to the study. Ask, for example, about the patient's main concern or chief complaint, health status, age, ethnicity, race, gender, and current treatment. Identifying the *intervention* is the second step in the PICO process. It is important to identify the treatment or intervention that will be used; for example, a new medication, a new method of brushing teeth, a new therapy, or a new procedure. The *comparison* is the main alternative treatment, and it can be a different intervention, usual care, or nothing at all. The *outcome* is the final component of the PICO format. It describes the intended or anticipated results, and it should be measurable. Outcomes can include relief of specific symptoms, such as pain, a decrease in length of stay, or decrease in infection. Outcomes should be as specific as possible. The PICO for the Americans-with-obesity question could be:

P = Obese Hispanic children between the ages of 13 and 17 years

I = A culturally congruent diet plan

C = Usual meal plan

O = A decease in body mass index (BMI) by 10%

The key components can now be stated as a question: *In obese Hispanic children, aged 13 through 17 years, what is the effect of a culturally congruent dietary plan on BMI?*

A PICO and its research question can also be qualitative. In such a case, PICO is referred to as PICo for population, interest phenomenon, and context. For example: What is the meaning of retirement (I) among elderly women (P) in an adult residential community (Co)? Another mnemonic that can be used for both quantitative and qualitative question development is SPICE: setting, perspective, intervention, comparison, and evaluation.

To determine whether this is a good clinical question, FINER (feasible, interesting, novel, ethical, relevant) questions can be asked. According to Cummings, Browner, and Hulley (2007), FINER questions include:

- Feasible

  Are there enough subjects? A preliminary calculation of sample size can be beneficial. There are a number of free online calculators that can help determine an adequate sample size (e.g., G-Power). If the calculated number of subjects seems too large, a number of strategies can be used, including expanding the inclusion criteria, lengthening the study's time frame, or recruiting another site into the study. Is the technical expertise available to conduct the study? Is the study affordable in time and money? Is the study manageable in scope?

- Interesting

  Are there others in addition to the researcher who find the question interesting? The researcher should speak with mentors, advisors, or outside experts or funding agencies before developing a project around a topic that others consider tedious.

- Novel

  Does the study confirm, extend, or refute a previous study?

- Ethical
     Is the study amenable to institutional review board guidelines? If a study has unacceptable physical or emotional risks or invades privacy, it should not be conducted. The researcher will need to seek other ways to investigate the topic.

- Relevant
     Is the study relevant to practice, policy, or further research? How will the findings of the study inform or advance practice, policy, or guide research?

APPROACHES TO SCHOLARLY INQUIRY

Scholarly inquiry takes one of three approaches: quantitative, qualitative, or mixed method; that is, a combination of the two approaches (see Table 2.2). The choice of a strategy for inquiry is dependent on the focus of the study. Is the focus an in-depth understanding (qualitative), a need to infer cause and effect (quantitative), or both (mixed method)?

TABLE 2.2 Qualitative Versus Quantitative Approaches to Inquiry

Characteristic	Quantitative	Qualitative
Purpose	Prediction, control, description, confirmation, hypothesis testing	Understanding of social phenomena through words and pictures
	Generalizability	Interpretation
Focus	Precise, but narrow outcomes	Holistic process
Design	Predetermined	Emergent
Tools	Instruments (scales, tests, surveys, questionnaires, computers)	The human person
Data	Objective	Subjective
Conditions	Artificial	Naturalistic
Advantages	Unbiased	More in-depth description of events, feelings, perceptions, experiences
Disadvantages	Lacks in-depth information	Study may lack reliability and validity
		Potential for researcher bias
Researcher role	Detached	Personal involvement

Qualitative inquiry is a general term for research methods, such as ethnography, grounded theory, phenomenology, or participant observation research. It emphasizes the importance of the natural setting. Exhaustive data are gathered through interviews using open-ended questions that provide direct quotations. The interviewer is an integral part of the investigation and is considered a research tool. This differs from the quantitative approach, which gathers data by objective methods, such as surveys or physiological measurements, to provide information about effects, associations, comparisons, and predictions. The investigator is remote from the data.

A qualitative approach is constructivist in nature (experiential thinking), and collects open-ended, emerging data with the intent of developing themes. Qualitative research uses detailed descriptions from the perspective of the research participants as a means of examining a phenomenon. The qualitative method is about exploring issues, perceptions, feelings and experiences, and understanding social phenomenon. It is also nonstatistical. Qualitative inquiry is an inductive process in which themes and categories emerge from the data. Samples are usually small, often less than 10, and are often purposively selected. Purposive sampling is an essential feature of qualitative inquiry in which subjects are selected based on some characteristics, such as gender, ethnicity, or having a certain condition, such as asthma. For example, a researcher may be interested in the at-home experiences of elderly Medicare beneficiaries with heart failure who are readmitted within 90 days of discharge from an acute care facility. The usual procedure in a qualitative study is to:

- Write the research question and select a qualitative strategy of inquiry
- Identify the researcher role
- Describe the selection-and-assignment process of participants
- Specify methods of collecting and recording of data
- Identify the steps in analyzing and coding the qualitative data to generate themes

A quantitative approach is one in which the scholar takes a primarily postpositive view to develop knowledge (reductionist thinking), collect data using surveys or other instruments that yield data for statistical analysis, and analyze the collected data using statistical techniques. Quantitative inquiry is about measurement, such as attitudes, satisfaction, laboratory values, physiological parameters, and anything that can be reduced to a number. Quantitative research tests theory. For example, what are the most important factors that influence a patient's choice of a primary care provider? The usual procedure for a quantitative study is to:

- Write the research question and identify the type of design
- Identify the population and sample
- Describe the recruitment, selection, and assignment process of participants
- Identify the instrument and report validity and reliability
- Specify the major variables
- Provide definition of terms
- Identify how validity is addressed in the design
- Describe the statistical tests to be used for data analysis

A mixed-method approach is a combination of qualitative and quantitative approaches. A rationale is developed for mixing the types of data at each stage of the inquiry (Creswell, 2003).

The decision as to which of the approaches to use is based on the type of question to be asked. It is important to clarify the type of question you are asking so that the best research design can be used. Types of questions can be categorized as therapy (i.e., treatment, interventions), diagnosis (i.e., the selection and interpretation of diagnostic tests), etiology (i.e., causation), prognosis (i.e., the effect or impact of a disease or condition), harm (consequences of disease or treatment), or meaning (see Table 2.3).

REFLECTIVE CRITIQUE

An essential activity in developing as a scholar is to reflect, critically, on one's work, both in terms of process and outcomes. The essential question to ask is: "What would I do differently next time?" In addition, the following questions can guide a reflective critique.

- How can I use the results of this project to improve my practice?
- What will I do next in terms of researching this topic?
- What facilitated my work?
- What challenges were encountered and were they amicably resolved?

TABLE 2.3   Suggested Designs to Answer Questions

Type of Question	Study Design
Therapy	Randomized controlled trials
	Nonrandomized trials
	Cohort study
	Case-control study
Diagnosis/Screening	Randomized controlled trials
	Nonrandomized trials
	Cohort study
	Case-control study
Etiology	Controlled trials
	Cohort study
Prognosis	Randomized controlled trials
	Nonrandomized trials
	Cohort study
	Case-control study
Harm	Randomized controlled trials
	Nonrandomized trials
	Cohort study
	Case-control study
Meaning	Case study
	Ethnography
	Grounded theory
	Action research
	Phenomenology

WRITING THE PROPOSAL

The purpose of writing a proposal for research is to provide a blueprint or plan of action that is predetermined. In this way, once the study is under way, the researcher need only look at the proposal and follow the procedures as described. The ideas presented in the proposal must flow logically and build on one another; in other words, the researcher builds a case for the study (Burns & Grove, 2009). An outline of essential components of a research proposal is presented in Box 2.1. Every proposal should contain the following:

Box 2.1

ESSENTIAL COMPONENTS OF A PROPOSAL

Introduction
Identify the focus of the study
Establish the significance of the study
Discuss one or two background studies related to the topic
State the study aims and research question
Explain how the study is relevant to nursing practice

Review of the Literature
Synthesize the literature on the topic
Summarize how the study will contribute to nursing knowledge by filling in gaps, validating, or testing knowledge

Theoretical Framework
Describe the theoretical framework to be used in the study
Connect the study aims and research questions to the theoretical framework
Operationally define study variables
Provide any study assumptions

Method
Describe the study design
Describe the setting and sample for the study, including inclusion and exclusion criteria
Describe how the sample will be recruited, if appropriate
Describe human subject protection methods
Describe how data will be collected, including the validity and reliability of any instruments to be used
Describe how data will be measured
State anticipated findings
State the limitations of the study

Time Frame
Describe the time it will take to complete the study
Provide a week-by-week listing of activities from start to completion

An *introduction* that provides an opening statement to demonstrate why this is an important area of inquiry is essential. The purpose of the study is stated and information on the background of the clinical problem and its significance are presented. Some statistics can be used to demonstrate the importance of the topic. This section should also contain the research question, the aims of the study, and a statement on why it is necessary to investigate this issue.

A *review of the literature* is the next step in writing a proposal. Salient articles should be located, critically analyzed, and synthesized. This section should describe the current state of knowledge about the topic. An explanation of how the proposed project or study will expand or validate knowledge should be included. This section is not an annotated bibliography but rather a thoughtful synthesis of current and relevant literature on the topic.

A *theoretical framework* provides an opportunity to connect the study aims and research question to a scaffold. A theory is a body of knowledge that organizes, describes, predicts, and/or explains phenomena (Fleury & Sidani, 2012). Theory that guides advanced practice should be testable, and include an "integrated set of concepts, existence statements, relational statements, and the expected changes in outcomes" (Fleury & Sidani, 2012, p. 12). Variables should be operationally defined within the context of the theory being used, and any study assumptions should be provided. It may be useful to draw a visual map depicting the relationships among the theories, concepts and propositions, and study variables.

A *method* section that outlines methods and procedures of the study is important and should be as clear and transparent as possible. It is necessary to have precise detail in explaining how the data answer the project question. The study design and a justification for its use should be included. The setting, sample (including inclusion and exclusion criteria), recruitment strategies, and how human subjects will be protected need to be described. The method of data analysis should be explained as well as a rationale as to why the specific methods of analysis were chosen.

It may be helpful to include a description of the intended outcomes and a timeline for completion so that the project stays on target.

CONCLUSION

Scholarship is defined as the discovery, integration, application, and teaching of knowledge. To be recognized as scholarship, activities must be guided by a focused clinical question, informed by current knowledge in the field, and follow established methods. Most important, it must be shared with others.

Engaging in scholarly inquiry around advanced nursing practice involves commitment, leadership, acceptance of challenges, and integration of evidence into practice. This includes those activities that are "(1) significant to the profession, (2) creative, (3) can be documented, (4) can be replicated or elaborated, and (5) can be peer-reviewed through various methods" (AACN, 1999, para. 5). Additionally, there is a responsibility for the advanced practice nurse to not only observe, describe, understand, and assess clinical phenomena through theoretical and empirical knowledge, but also to translate best evidence and evaluate the impact on health outcomes (Margery, Whitney, & Brown, 2006).

REFLECTIVE EXERCISES

1. Rewrite the following questions into their PICO components. Then determine the FINER criteria for each one:
   - What is the relationship between depression and delirium?
   - Does eating fish contribute to a healthier heart?
   - Can simulated experiences increase self-confidence?
   - Does pet therapy decrease length of stay?
   - Does increased intravenous fluid work when treating patients with severe burns?
2. Think about your advanced practice situation. What areas do you think need further investigation? What theoretical framework will inform the investigation?

REFERENCES

American Association of Colleges of Nursing. (1999). Defining scholarship for the discipline of nursing. *Proceedings of the AACN Task Force on Defining Standards for the Scholarship of Nursing.* Washington, DC: Author.

Boyer, E. L. (1990). *Scholarship reconsidered: Priorities of the professoriate.* Princeton, NJ: Carnegie Foundation for the Advancement of Teaching.

Burns, N., & Grove, S. (2009). *The practice of nursing research.* Philadelphia, PA: Saunders.

Creswell, J. (2003). *Research design: Qualitative, quantitative and mixed method approaches.* Thousand Oaks, CA: Sage.

Cummings, S., Browner, W., & Hulley, S. (2007). Conceiving the research question. In S. Hulley, S. Cummings, W. Browner, D. Grady, & T. Newman (Eds.), *Designing clinical research* (3rd ed., pp. 18–26). Philadelphia, PA: Lippincott Williams & Wilkins.

Fleury, J., & Sidani, S. (2012). Using theory to guide intervention research. In B. Melnyk & D. Morrison-Beedy (Eds.), *Intervention research.* New York, NY: Springer Publishing Company.

Kitchenham, B. (2004). *Procedures for systematic reviews: Joint technical report.* Retrieved from http://www.ask.com/web?gct=serp&qsrc=2417&o=100000 031&l=dis&locale=en_US&tpr=2&q=Kitchenham+and+systematic+review

Margary, D., Whitney, J., & Brown, M. (2006). Advancing practice inquiry: Research foundations of the doctor of nursing practice. *Nursing Outlook, 54*(3), 139–142.

SUGGESTED READING

American Association of Colleges of Nursing. (1999). Defining scholarship for the discipline of nursing. *Proceedings of the AACN Task Force on Defining Standards for the Scholarship of Nursing.* Washington, DC: Author. Retrieved from http://www.aacn.nche.edu/publications/position/defining-scholarship

Cummings, S., Browner, W., & Hulley, S. (2007). *Conceiving the research question.* Retrieved from http://spctrm.stanford.edu/education/ICCR2011/ Mod01-Lavori_ConceivingtheResearchQuestion_M1.pdf

Morrison, C. (2012). 'Boyer reconsidered': Fostering students' scholarly habits of mind and models of practice. *International Journal for the Scholarship of Teaching and Learning, 6*(1), 1–15. Retrieved from http://www.georgiasouthern.edu/ ijsotl

Methods of Scholarship

Action Research

OBJECTIVES

At the end of this chapter, you will be able to:
- Define action research
- Explain the process of action research
- Select a clinical problem suitable for action research
- Define the role of the action research facilitator

KEY CONCEPTS

- Action research directly impacts practice.

- An aim of action research is to build capacity.

- Action research is a cycle of data collection, reflection, and problem redefinition.

- Action research uses a variety of qualitative and quantitative methods to collect data, although words are more important than numbers.

- Action research is a community of practice.

Action research is a reflective process about research in action. It is grounded in context, and involves real-world situations and problems. It is a constantly evolving method of inquiry conducted within familiar settings by teams working together for the resolution of practice problems. The personal familiarity of the researchers with the research setting confers relevance and credibility to both the inquiry process and its findings. In other words, it is done by and with insiders, those central to and conversant with the areas to be researched (Herr & Anderson, 2005). Rather than dwelling on the theoretical, action research allows practitioners to address those real-life concerns over which they can exhibit some influence and have the ability and authority to make needed change (Ferrance, 2000). However, some amount of knowledge is always gained through action, which implies that action research is also empirical in its processes. Experimental research, for example, is about manipulation and control using causal models. In action research, there is not the same level of control when interventions are initiated. The researcher uses observation and interviews as key data-collection approaches. For example, Alyward, Murphy, Colmer, and O'Neill (2010) observed and interviewed parents over an 18-month period to determine the success of an intervention targeted toward parents of children aged birth to 5 years with attachment issues.

Reason and Bradbury (2007) refer to action research as a "democratic process concerned with developing practical knowledge" (p. 1). Action research is known by a variety of other names as well (Table 3.1), although for the purposes of this chapter, the term *action research* will be used. In essence, action research is a deliberate, solution-oriented investigation characterized by a circular process of problem identification, data collection, analysis, reflection, data-derived action, evaluation, further reflection, and problem redefinition (Kemmis & McTaggart, 1992). The underlying principle is one of change and redirection as determined by continual reflection on data gathered and actions taken, and proceeding through the cycle as many times as necessary to find a solution (Figure 3.1). It is not the linear approach attributed to the scientific method. In this sense, action research resembles the nursing process

TABLE 3.1 Synonyms for Action Research

Action research

Participatory action research

Community-based action research

Community-of-practice research

Cooperative inquiry

Practitioner research

Collaborative research

Appreciative inquiry

Action science

Cooperative inquiry

Developmental-action inquiry

Praxis intervention

Community-engaged research

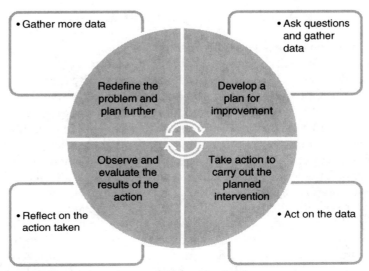

FIGURE 3.1   The Cyclical Nature of Action Research

and its steps of assessing, planning, implementing, evaluating, and re-planning (Glasson, Chang, & Bidewell, 2008).

As illustration, suppose that an investigation was conducted within an acute care hospital to examine the increasing number of patients being held in the emergency department (ED) who were awaiting beds. A group consisting of the ED nursing and medical directors, ED administrator, two ED staff nurses, and one ED physician meet to examine the issue more closely, and write a report based on their examination. Can that research be considered action research if the report based on it is used by the hospital administration to initiate a process that allows better patient flow through the department and the hospital as a whole? The answer is "yes" if the research report is used to initiate change, and allows for a follow-up evaluation of the impact of that change, and if those in charge of ED flow are involved in the process. The answer is "no" if the research ended with a report of the investigation sitting on someone's desk or discussed at a meeting with little or no change in processes. In other words, "Action research is not merely research which it is hoped will be followed by action! It is action which is intentionally researched and modified leading to the next stage of action which is then again intentionally examined for further change and soon is a part of the search itself" (Wadsworth, 1998, p. 3).

ACTION RESEARCH

The term *action research* was first used in 1946 by Kurt Lewin to describe the process of investigating intergroup relationships in the United States (Reason & Rowan, 1981). Lewin described it as research that did not separate the investigation from the action needed to solve the problem (Ferrance, 2000). The strength of action research, according to Meyer (2000), lies in both its ability to generate practical solutions to real-life problems and build capacity among practitioners as they develop and implement activities to solve the identified problem. Action research is a collection of research methodologies used to pursue action (or change) and research (or knowledge) at the same time. Thus, the researchers are directly involved in the practice that is being researched (Ferrance, 2000), and practitioners are directly involved in the research that is being conducted. Action research is based primarily on the assumption that practitioners, at immediate and concrete levels, are best able to identify, understand, and find solutions for practice problems (Table 3.2).

THE PRINCIPLES OF ACTION RESEARCH

Democracy

The representative nature of action research may be one of its greatest benefits as it grounds the research process in real-world practice. Academic researchers and clinical practice experts work together as equals to determine the problem, the action, its process for change, and the way in which it will be implemented and evaluated (Meyer, 2000). Hierarchal differences are flattened. For example, a team of researchers, prison officials, and inmates convened inside a women's maximum security prison to investigate the impact of offering access to higher education to inmates, ultimately documenting that education

TABLE 3.2 Assumptions Underlying Action Research

Practitioners are best able to understand practice problems in need of a solution.

Change and redirection as needed are essential to action research.

Practice itself is a form of research as one attempts various ways to obtain good outcomes.

To be excellent, a practitioner needs to engage in substantial reflection about the nature of practice.

Collaboration among teams of health care providers is crucial for process improvement.

for prisoners can change communities, reduce crime, and save taxpayer dollars (Torre & Fine, 2005). This is not an easy process. As Prilleltensky (1997) tells us, it is necessary not only to be able to talk about the values of a democratic relationship but to be able to apply these concepts in action. In the prison study, the inmates were equal in participation and voice to the prison officials. Smith and colleagues (2010) relate the experiences of a gay White male graduate student working on an action research project with inner-city gay homeless teens. At the first collaborative meeting, the graduate student was asked to share who he was and why he was there. Despite having discussed this same question with the outside research group, he reflected:

> in the moment that I was asked to participate in that same discussion with participants, I was struck with an anxiety-provoking realization. It was easy to say to my colleagues at school that I wanted to help and advocate for queer youth in our city. However, to say "I want to help you" to a group of people who were actually more comfortable with their sexuality than I was seemed incredibly presumptuous. Immediately, I realized that I was still not viewing the organization's members as equal partners in the project. (p. 412)

According to Stringer (2007), participation in action research is built on the key concepts of significant levels of active involvement, performance of specific tasks, support for each other as participants learn about each other and the problem at hand, setting goals that can be achieved within a certain time frame, and face-to-face discussion with stakeholders, rather than through representatives.

Feedback

Throughout an action research project, findings are given back to participants for validation and to inform decisions about the next stage of the study. This formative style of research is responsive to events as they in the field and frequently requires iterations of reflection, action, and re-reflection. Feedback should be information specific, issue focused, and based on observations. The purpose of such feedback is to determine how successful events to improve a process have been and to outline the next steps.

All relevant stakeholders should be provided the necessary feedback on a regular basis. Feedback strategies should be a part of the overall approach to the project and can include regularly scheduled meetings, prearranged visits, telephone calls, or project updates sent by e-mail. According to Stringer (2007), it is important that "each person be linked with others so that participants can discuss their problems, celebrate accomplishments, maintain focus, and sustain their sense of identity with the project" (p. 134).

Multiple Goals

Action research is characterized by first-, second-, and third-person research goals. In the first person, one's own actions are researched for the purposes of personal change. Second-person research is aimed at ways to improve the group (or community or family). Third-person research is scholarly research aimed primarily at theoretical generalization and/ or large-scale change. Goals for each of these agendas are possible within an action research framework. For example, in a research study with the objective of improving the care of older people at risk of delirium, nursing staff wanted experience doing research (first person). They were motivated by the idea of being active participants in developing and implementing improved patient-care processes that could reduce the risk of delirium in older people (second person), and also wanted to evaluate management guidelines and establish quality-monitoring criteria for this group of patients (third person; Li et al., 2010).

CHARACTERISTICS OF ACTION RESEARCH

One of the key characteristics that distinguishes action research from most other research approaches, and also constitutes one of its main appeals, is that action research aims at both improving a process and generating knowledge, and achieving both at the same time (Kock, 2011). As Meyer (2000) points out, action research "is an approach which demands that participants perceive the need to change and are willing to play an active part in the research and the change process" (p. 178). This level of participation requires a commitment that goes beyond simply collecting data or answering questions. Active participation by stakeholders in the process is crucial to its success. The goals of action research, according to Herr and Anderson (2005), involve generating new knowledge, attaining action-oriented outcomes that are relevant to the setting, and educating team members using a sound research method. To achieve these goals, action research must establish key indicators of performance, which can be used as audit criteria as the project unfolds. Key performance indicators are metrics regarding how well goals are being met. There is no set standard for the development of indicators, but there should be at least one indicator for each project goal. Well-developed indicators are relevant, clearly defined, and easily measured (National Institute for Health and Clinical Excellence [NICE], 2002).

Action research appeals to nurses due to its success in systems improvement and patient outcomes (Badger, 2000), as well as its ability to narrow the theory–practice gap (Rolfe, 1996). Suitable subjects for action research are those that "(a) are real events, which must be managed in real time, (b) provide opportunities for both effective action and learning, and (c) can contribute to the development of theory of what really goes on in hospitals and to the development of nursing knowledge" (Coghlan & Casey, 2001, p. 675). Examples suitable for action research include:

- An examination of the use of shared medical equipment
- A process to decrease 30-day readmissions among home care patients
- The transition from an intensive care unit to a general nursing unit
- The development of a procedure for therapeutic hypothermia
- A process to address high suicide rates among adolescents
- Installation of new computer systems, such as electronic health records
- Determining the effects of a new teaching strategy

Once the notions of traditional research are swept away, the essential characteristics of action research are fairly straightforward. Reflection during each phase of the action cycle is crucial to success. Those involved must recollect and then critique what has already happened. The increased understanding that emerges from this reflection is then put to use in designing the next steps. For example, in the ED waiting-time study, the action research team first needed to understand the extent and nature of the waiting-time problem. They began by a general discussion of the issue and how it impacted each of their individual role functions and patient and family satisfaction. Next, they decided they needed more specific data and set up a process to review the medical records of those patients who waited longer than 30 minutes in the ED.

FRAMEWORKS FOR ACTION RESEARCH

Action research is an intentional method that involves (*Nursing Planet*, 2011):

- Marking very clear statements about the clinical issue
- Developing goals for improvement

- Formulating action plans to meet the goals
- Observing the effects of the actions
- Reflecting on the observations
- Re-planning based on reflections

Yet, the use of various terms to refer to action research (Table 3.1) implies that the concept of action research has different meanings to different people, which can lead to very different definitions and forms of practice (Hinchey, 2008). Dewey (1916), for example, believed that all research should be done by those central to the issue, rather than by outsiders. He argued that those in the field needed to do the testing involved in developing practices. Others, such as Heron (1997), posited that cooperative inquiry, or collaborative inquiry, is the basis of action research and that the research is conducted *with* people, rather than *on* people. All participants in the process are considered coresearchers.

Freire (2000) believed that action research is participatory, and that even students can be participants in research on their own learning as they construct their own knowledge. In what he called participatory action research (PAR), people are empowered to bring change by generating knowledge through reflection on personal experiences and

TABLE 3.3   Some Sources of Data for Action Research

Qualitative	Quantitative
Interviews	Surveys
Portfolios	Records
Diaries	Reports
Field notes	Attendance
Audiotapes	Self-assessment
Photos	
Memos	
Questionnaires	
Focus groups	
Anecdotal records	
Journals	
Individual files	
Logs of meetings	
Videotapes	
Case studies	

situations (Glasson, Change, & Bidwell, 2008). For example, in a study of palliative care, the practitioner-researchers shared practice stories and analyzed these stories to identify practice issues, such as clinical judgment, the way people die, not being able to provide care, and misunderstandings of palliative nursing (Taylor et al., 2008).

Torbert and Trullen (2004) believed that action inquiry demands attention to what is occurring at the personal, group, and organizational levels in the midst of the action, which allows for immediate learning and understanding of the area being researched.

Kemmis and McTaggert (1998) define action research as a form of collective inquiry undertaken by participants in social situations to improve their own practice as well as their understanding of those practices and the situations in which these practices are carried out.

To summarize the common understanding among these action-research frameworks: Real-world practice challenges need analysis and action and re-analysis; the results are shared with the larger community for critique and evaluation; stakeholders are identified early in the process and collectively agree on the problem to be addressed; all participants in the action research project are coresearchers; and reflecting on the process and results throughout the project is an important action to be taken by all involved.

DATA COLLECTION

Action research primarily draws from qualitative methods of data collection, although the specific methods used are dependent on the question asked and the problem under investigation (see Table 3.3). Most important, when conducting an action research project, baseline data are needed so that improvement can be documented as a result of action taken. Some of the more common methods used to collect data for an action research study are listed here.

Focus groups, as the name implies, engage in targeted or focused discussion about issues, actions, or outcomes significant to the research project. Those representative of the stakeholders in the project are convened for this interview. Focus groups are useful in developing a more in-depth understanding of a particular issue than could occur at a project meeting with a wide-ranging agenda. Focus group questions can be structured, semistructured, or unstructured, depending on the topic for discussion. A researcher might ask only predetermined questions in a structured interview to ensure that specific questions are answered, a useful and efficient strategy when the researcher is clear about exactly what he or she wants to know. However, "less structured interviews hold the possibility of expanding the researcher's thinking; given free rein to shape the conversation, a participant following his own line of thinking may open a new perspective the researcher hadn't considered" (Hinchey, 2011, p. 11). Construction of questions is an important pre-focus group activity as the researcher does not want to influence the participants' answers. For example, the question, "Would you agree that this policy is depriving our staff of needed resources?" calls for a very different response than "Do you have any thoughts on how this policy has affected staff satisfaction?"

Field notes are records written by the researcher about ongoing events that occur during the study. Hinchey (2011) explains that notes can be written in a number of ways, such as sweeping notes (a recording every 5 minutes), event notes (a record of all events during an observation), critical incident notes (a recording of crucial points in a study), or summary notes (written at the end of an event or day). Field notes typically are in the form of a diary or journal that provides a record of the chronological events and the researcher's reflection on activities and his or her own opinions on the progress of the project.

Surveys are questionnaires used to gather data from many people. Very focused questions are important to this method. For example, "Do you give medications to your patients daily?" is too broad when you want to know the number of medication episodes. Free online-survey software such as Survey Monkey (www.surveymonkey.com) can be used effectively as it allows for anonymity and multiple types of question formats.

Documents might need to be reviewed to gain an enlarged understanding of the problem under study. Documents important to most process change include meeting minutes, policies, procedures, statistical reports, or quality-improvement (including accreditation) reports. If the action research study is concerned with an education issue, documents such as student papers, course evaluations, and student handbooks are also important.

Observation of the processes under study is also common. Observations can be counted (e.g., the number of times a nurse is interrupted when passing medication), measured in time (e.g., the length of time for a bedside report), or described (e.g., the interaction among surgeons and nurses in the operating room). Observation is often combined with interviewing. Interviewing participants can provide a greater understanding and rationale for activities or behaviors that have been observed. Typically, the observer takes on a passive data-collection role, using a checklist or writing field notes. Audio and video recording may also be used, although this would require additional institutional review board review and focused informed consents.

THE CHALLENGES OF ACTION RESEARCH

Action research is not without its challenges. Commitment to the project, which may take a number of months to complete, determination of data ownership, and budget are important issues that need to be discussed in the planning stages of the project.

The Challenge of Commitment

The level of commitment required in an action research study goes beyond simply taking part in a meeting, completing a survey, or agreeing to be observed. Core features of action research are that the work happens in the context of action partnership with practitioners. Not only must practitioners see the value of working with researchers, they must want to engage in the research process. Action researchers need to plan both for cycles of action and time for reflection so that practitioners see the value in what they are doing and remain committed (Bradbury, 2010).

The Challenge of Democracy

In action research, participants are equals as hierarchal differences are flattened (Mendenhall & Doherty, 2005). The researcher works as a facilitator of change, consulting with clinical site practitioners not only on the action process but also on how it will be evaluated, which roots the investigation in everyday practice. Findings are shared and discussed at each stage of the process and used to inform decisions about the next stage. This developmental style of research is thus responsive to naturally occurring clinical events in real time. However, as Meyer (2000) points out, care needs to be taken as the democratic process may be threatened because it is not a usual feature of health care settings. An action researcher needs to be able to work across traditional boundaries (e.g., between health and social work professionals or between hospital and community care settings) and juggle different, sometimes competing, agendas. This requires excellent interpersonal skills as well as research ability. As Brown, Bammer, Baltiwala, and Kunreuther (2003) point out, "practitioners bring (their own) frameworks . . . with their own definitions of excellence and effectiveness" (p. 89); therefore, researchers need to be aware of the potential need to renegotiate goals (Reed, 2005).

The Challenge of Process

Simultaneous gathering and acting on data to influence practice may be a challenge as this lends itself not only to the discovery of solutions, but also to the uncovering of new or unknown clinical issues. It can be a "slow and messy process," especially in the early phases of the research (Mendelhall & Doherty, 2005). Care needs to be taken to remain on target through development of short- and long-term goals and discussion of these at team meetings. In this regard, a project leader skilled in facilitation is needed. Facilitation is a technique in which the actions of one person make the work of others easier. Facilitation moves along a range of activities that are both task focused (e.g., project management) and enabling (e.g., personal development; Kitson et al., 2008). The facilitator offers change strategies, supports the process, and provides support in the analysis of data. A facilitator needs to be cognizant of the influence of the organizational culture and other influences that may interfere with naturalistic inquiries and make plans to ease these influences (Holly et al., 2013).

WRITING THE ACTION RESEARCH REPORT

Overall, the final report for an action research study is similar to the standard research report format with study purpose, literature review, methods, results, discussion, and conclusions. The additional elements needed in an action research report include:

- A description of the context, which includes descriptions of the organizational structure, stakeholders, and patients served
- An explanation of how the clinical problem was determined to be a problem in need of action along with the goals of the project and their key indicators of performance
- A description that focuses on how the clinical problem was investigated prior to the start of the project. Included here should be the viewpoints of those knowledgeable about the clinical problem using their own words, rather than the usual, more objective research-presentation voice, plus any available baseline data.
- A description of the role and responsibilities of each of the team members, including the project facilitator

CONCLUSION

In summary, action research tends to be participative (researchers and clinicians are involved as process partners), cyclic (steps in the process are sequential and spiral), qualitative (dealing more with language than numbers), and reflective (thinking about the process and redefining and re-planning for each cycle). See Table 3.4 for a sample of resources for action researchers.

TABLE 3.4 Online Resources for Action Research

General Resources

  Action Research in the Americas

    sites.google.com/site/arnaconnect

  Center for Collaborative Action Research

    cadres.pepperdine.edu/ccar

  Online source for action research

    www.lupinworks.com/ar/index.html

For Educators

  Action Research at Queen's University

    resources.educ.queensu.ca/ar

  Action Research in Education

    www.edu.plymouth.ac.uk/resined/actionresearch/arhome.htm

Health Care

  Action Research in Nursing

    nursingplanet.com/Nursing_Research/action_research_nursing.html

  Carrying Out Action Research on Health Interventions

    www.microinsurancefacility.org/en/learning-journey/bringing-%E2%80%
    9Chealth%E2%80%9D-health-insurance-evidence-converged-approach/
    project-lessons/carr

REFLECTIVE EXERCISES

Reflect on a practice problem that you believe is in need of a solution. Plan your approach:

1. What do you hope to accomplish?
2. What baseline data do you need to fully understand the problem? Where will these data come from?
3. Who will be members of your team?
4. Do you need a champion?
5. Who will you have to convince that change is needed?

REFERENCES

Aylward, P., Murphy, P., Colmer, K., & O'Neill, M. (2010). Findings from an evaluation of an intervention targeting Australian parents of young children with attachment issues: The 'Through the Looking Glass' (TtLG) project. *Australasian Journal of Early Childhood, 35*(3), 13–23.

Badger, T. G. (2000). Action research, change and methodological rigour. *Journal of Nursing Management, 8*, 201–207.

Bradbury, H. H. (2010). What is good action research. *Action Research, 8*(1), 93–109.

Brown, D. L., Bammer, G., Baltiwala, S., & Kunreuther, F. (2003). Framing practice-research engagement for democratizing knowledge. *Action Research, 1*, 81–102.

Coghan, D., & Casey, M. (2001). Action research from the inside: Issues and challenges in doing action research in your own hospital. *Journal of Advanced Nursing, 35*(5), 674–682.

Dewey, J. (1916). *Democracy and education*. New York, NY: The Free Press. Retrieved from http://books.google.com/books/about/Democracy_and_Education.html?id=19ajcXf4MCYC

Ferrance, E. (2000). *Themes in education: Action research*. Providence, RI: Northeast and Regional Educational Laboratory at Brown University.

Freire, P. (2000). *Pedagogy of the oppressed* (30th Anniversary ed.). New York, NY: Continuum Press.

Glasson, J., Chang, E., & Bidewell, J. (2008). The value of participatory action research in clinical nursing practice. *International Journal of Nursing Practice, 14*(1), 34–39.

Heron, J. (1997). *Co-operative inquiry: Research into the human condition*. Thousand Oaks, CA: Sage.

Herr, K., & Anderson, G. L. (2005). *The action research dissertation*. Thousand Oaks, CA: Sage.

Hinchey, P. (2008). *Action research primer*. New York, NY: Peter Lang Publishing.

Holly, C., Percy, M., Salmond, S., Caldwell, B., Echevarria, M., & Bugel, M. J. (2013). *When cultures collide: Academic and clinical teams join forces to move evidence into practice*. Unpublished manuscript. Newark, NJ: University of Medicine and Dentistry of NJ, School of Nursing. Retrieved from hollych@rutgers.edu

Kemmis, S., & McTaggart, R. (1992). *The action research reader* (3rd ed.). Waurn Ponds, Australia: Deakin University Press.

Kitson, A., Rycroft-Malone, J., Harvey, G., McCormack, B., Seers, K., & Titchen, A. (2008). Evaluating the successful implementation of evidence into practice using the PARiHS Framework: Theoretical and practical challenges. *Implementation Science, 3*(1). Retrieved from www.implementationscience.com/content/3/1/1

Kock, N. (2011). Action research: Its nature and relationship to human-computer interaction. In M. Soegaard & R. F. Dam (Eds.), *Encyclopedia of human-computer interaction*. Retrieved from www.interaction design.org/encyclopedia/action_research.html

Li, P., Bashford, L., Schwager, G., Spain, R., Ryan, H., Oakman, M., . . . Higgins, I. (2010). Clinicians' experiences of participating in an action research study. *Contemporary Nurse, 35*(2), 147–156.

Mendenhall, T., & Doherty, W. (2005). Action research methods in family therapy. In F. Piercy & D. Sprenkle (Eds.), *Research methods in family therapy* (2nd ed., pp. 100–117). New York, NY: Guilford Press.

Meyer, J. (2000). Using qualitative methods in health related action research. *British Medical Journal, 3206*, 178.

National Institute for Health and Clinical Excellence. (2002). *Principles for best practice in clinical audit.* Oxford, England: Radical Medical Press.

Nursing Planet. (2011). *Action research in nursing.* Retrieved from http://nursing planet.com/Nursing_Research/action_research_nursing.html

Prilleltensky, I. (1997). Values, assumptions, and practices: Assessing the moral implications of psychological discourse and action. *American Psychologist, 52*(5), 517–535.

Reason, P., & Bradbury, H. (2007). *Handbook of action research* (2nd ed.). London, England: Sage.

Reason, P., & Rowan, J. (1981). *Human inquiry: A sourcebook for paradigm research.* Chichester, England: Wiley.

Reed, J. (2005). Using action research in nursing practice with older people: Democratizing knowledge. *Journal of Clinical Nursing, 14*(5), 594–600.

Rolfe, G. (1996). Going to extremes: Action research, grounded practice and the theory–practice gap in nursing. *Journal of Advanced Nursing, 24*, 1315–1320.

Smith, L., Bratini, L., Chambers, D., Jensen, R., & Romero, L. (2010). Between idealism and reality: Meeting the challenges of participatory action research. *Action Research, 8*, 407–425.

Stringer, E. (2007). *Action research* (3rd ed.). Thousand Oaks, CA: Sage.

Taylor, B., Bewley, J., Bulmer, B., Hickey, A., Hill, L., Luxford, C., . . . Stirling, K. (2010). Getting it right under pressure: Action research and reflection in palliative nursing. *International Journal of Palliative Nursing, 14*(7), 326–331.

Torbert, W., & Turllen, J. (2004). First-, second-, and third-person research in practice. *Systems Thinker, 15*(1), 7–8.

Torre, M., & Fine, M. (2005). Bar none: Extending affirmative action to higher education in prison. *Journal of Social Issues, 61*(3), 569–594.

Wadsworth, Y. (1998). *What is participatory action research? Action Research International, paper 2.* Retrieved from www.scu.edu.au/schools/gcm/ar/ari/p-ywadsworth98.html

SUGGESTED READING

Coghan, D., & Casey, M. (2001). Action research from the inside: Issues and challenges in doing action research in your own hospital. *Journal of Advanced Nursing, 35*(5), 674–682.

Glasson, J., Chang, E., Chenoweth, L., Hancock, K., Hall, T., Hill-Murray, F., & Collier, L. (2006). Evaluation of a model of nursing care for older patients using participatory action research in an acute medical ward. *Journal of Clinical Nursing, 15*, 588–598.

Hope, K. W., & Waterman, H. A. (2003). Praiseworthy pragmatism: Validity and action research. *Journal of Advanced Nursing, 44*(2), 120–127.

Reed, J. (2005). Using action research in nursing practice with older people: Democratizing knowledge. *Journal of Clinical Nursing, 14*(5), 594–600.

Addressing the Use of Shared Medical Equipment in a Large Urban Hospital*

MARY JO BUGEL AND DENEEN SCUDERI

Background: Addressing infection-control issues is a top priority for health care organizations. The consequences of nonadherence to standard infection-control practices include poor patient outcomes and financial burdens to the organization. The research literature notes that there is a high prevalence of microorganisms, including epidemiologically significant, multidrug-resistant microorganisms in the patient care environment. These microorganisms are found in high concentrations on high-touch surfaces such as bedside tables, commodes, over-bed tables, bedrails, doorknobs, sinks and surfaces, and shared noncritical patient equipment. Stringent and frequent decontamination of these surfaces has shown to prevent transmission and curtail outbreaks. Even after routine cleaning of equipment, a level of bioburden remains on the surface. Although cleaning and disinfecting noncritical patient care equipment are included in standard precautions for infection prevention, the guidelines leave room for much interpretation.

* This project was part of a larger knowledge translation project called the Signature Project, a joint venture between the Rutgers School of Nursing (as University of Medicine and Dentistry of New Jersey School of Nursing) in Newark, New Jersey, USA, and the University of Adelaide School of Nursing in Adelaide, Australia, which involved four hospitals and one visiting nurse service. The assistance of the Signature Project team is acknowledged: University of Adelaide: Dr. Alison Kitson (PI), Dr. Richard Wiechula, Dr. Tim Schultz, Tiffany Conroy. UMDNJ Team: Dr. Cheryl Holly (site PI), Dr. Susan Salmon, Dr. Barbara Caldwell, Dr. Mary Jo Bugel, Dr. Melanie Percy, and Dr. Mercedes Echevarria.

Purpose: This project aimed to construct and implement a best-practice approach for the use and disinfection of noncritical portable medical devices to decrease equipment-related hospital-acquired infections (HAI). The most common portable equipment (glucometers and portable temperature units) were targeted.

Method: This is an action research study using pre- and postintervention observation and focus groups. The community of practice consisted of two nurse managers, the director of education, the director of infection control, and a nursing faculty member. The director of education served as the group facilitator to guide the team through identification and understanding of evidence, whereas the faculty member provided guidance in the use of the scientific method as (first person). The project was conducted on two inpatient units: a neonatal intensive care unit (ICU) and an adult medical–surgical unit in a large urban medical center.

Focus groups were held to determine current practice and identify barriers to the cleaning of shared noncritical patient equipment. Participants in the focus groups were the clinical staff providing patient care within these units who had first identified the issue; that is, the professional nurses and nursing assistants and staff from environmental services (second person). Baseline data for multidrug-resistant HAI rates for the medical–surgical and neonatal ICU were obtained. Observations were conducted by the infection-control practitioners using an observational data tool to determine how and if staff members were cleaning equipment between patient use and according to manufacturer's recommendations.

Adapting evidence to the local context, examining context for barriers to implementation, and developing a local plan of action to put evidence into action were major steps. A three-point plan was developed: education, policy and procedure revision, and a change in the location of disinfection supplies (second person).

Findings: Preinterventional data collection revealed equipment was not cleaned per manufacturer's recommendations 40.54% of the time; users could not identify whether equipment was clean 13.51% of the time; and equipment was visibly soiled 16.21% of the time. Postinterventional data collection revealed that users cleaned the equipment both before and after using 69.2% of the time. These findings were significant at less than $p = 0.05$. When equipment was cleaned, the correct cleaning agent was used according to manufacturer's instructions 100% of the time. When equipment was not cleaned, sanitizing solutions were not available 50% of the time.

One of the greatest contributors to staff not cleaning equipment identified during the focus group sessions was that sanitizing solutions were not readily available. In every instance staff identified the importance of cleaning equipment in between each patient use, demonstrating that there was not a lack of knowledge in this area. The lack of knowledge was that staff could not always identify the manufacturer's recommendations for proper cleaning of equipment. This was addressed by having a representative of the solution company conduct training sessions on the use of the solution.

Conclusion: Given the positive results of this action study in the identification and resolution of a clinical issue identified by front-line staff, the project will be implemented in all areas of the medical center (third person).

4

Case Study Research

OBJECTIVES

At the end of this chapter, you will be able to:
- Describe the key features of a case study
- Explain the components of a case study
- Explain the strategies for making meaning from case study data

KEY CONCEPTS

- Case study research brings a greater depth of understanding to complex issues through contextual analysis.
- A case study can be of an individual, a group (such as a family or hospital unit), an institution, or an entire community.
- Case study methodology is appropriate for describing, exploring, and understanding a phenomenon in its real-life context.
- A variety of data-collection methods are necessary.
- Case study research fits within the postpositive philosophy, meaning that there is thinking and reflection on what has happened after it happened.

A case study begins with a story about something special or interesting. The story is followed by an intensive analysis. Constructing a case study offers an opportunity to highlight success, to bring attention to a particular challenge or difficulty, or to describe a unique or unusual event. Cases might be selected because they are highly effective, not effective, representative, typical, or of special interest (Zucker, 2001). A case study is also an inquiry method that allows investigation of a clinical problem within a particular context bounded by time, place, and activity, and in which multiple sources of evidence are used (Yin, 1994, p. 23). As a research method, a case study can be used when the interaction among many factors needs to be understood. Case study research has been criticized as being unreliable and nongeneralizable because the number of cases studied is usually very small; in fact, one case can make a case study.

On the other hand, a case study describes real-life situations, issues, and problems, and provides an understanding as to how clinicians resolve issues or develop programs. "Thus, case studies comprise more detail, richness, completeness, and variance—that is, depth" than other types of research methods (Flyvbjerg, 2011, p. 301). The value of the case study lies in its invaluable descriptions of processes, interactions, and relationships. Such descriptions are phenomenologically distinctive and permit identification with the experience of the worker and the reality of the clinical encounter, albeit vicariously (Brandell & Varkas, 2001, p. 294).

The terms *case study*, *case review*, and *case report* are used synonymously; however, the key feature of a case study is that it is idiographic, meaning that the unit of study (or unit of analysis) is a single unit, and the unit can be an individual, team, family, community, organization, or process (Brandell & Varkas, 2001). A case study is a "systematic inquiry into an event or a set of related events which aims to describe and explain the phenomenon of interest" (Bromley, 1990, p. 302), with a defined focus and a specific time frame (Miles & Huberman, 1994). Case study research allows a deeper understanding of a complex issue or process and can add to what is already known. This is accomplished through a detailed contextual analysis of events or conditions and their relationships using documentation, archival records, interviews, direct observations, participant observation, and physical artifacts among other data-collection methods (Yin, 2009; Zucker, 2001). For example, case studies of individual patients often involve in-depth interviews with participants and key informants, review of the medical records, observation, and excerpts from patients' personal writings and diaries; whereas case studies of an organization or system involve review of meeting agendas and minutes, reports, and policies and procedures. Woodside (2010) maintains that using multiple methods such as these to triangulate confirms and deepens understanding, providing what Yin (2009) calls a chain of evidence.

A case study done for the purpose of examining phenomena is not the same as a case study used for teaching purposes in the classroom. Freud's case study of Dora is a famous example of the use of a case study to explain unusual symptoms that might be useful in similar situations (cubicle-notes.tripod.com/essays/id20.html). When using case studies for teaching application of theory, one is not concerned with rigor or empirical data (Yin, 2009). Conducting case study research implies that the researcher has a question and will use the scientific method to find an answer.

According to Yin (2009) a case study design should be used when: (a) the question guiding the study is a "how" and/or a "why" question, (b) the behavior of those involved in the study cannot be manipulated, (c) the context is important to the study, or (d) there are no clear boundaries between the unit of analysis and the context. See Table 4.1 for criteria for selecting

TABLE 4.1   Criteria for Selecting Cases

1. Extreme/deviant cases	To obtain information on unusual cases as a means of developing new concepts, variables, and theories related to the deviant cases.
2. Maximum-variation cases	To obtain information about the significance of process and outcome; e.g., cases that differ in size, organization, location, staffing, budget, etc.
3. Critical cases	To achieve information that permits logical deductions of the type, "If this is (not) valid for this case, then it applies to all (no) cases."
4. Paradigmatic cases	To develop a metaphor or establish a school for the domain that the case concerns.

Adapted from Flyvbjerg (2011).

a case study. For instance, in a study of pressure ulcer occurrence in the intensive care unit (ICU), Flike (2013) sought to determine if pressure ulcers could be prevented by using a specific protocol and assessment tool. A case study was chosen because the case was of a patient who developed a suspected deep tissue injury that progressed to a stage III pressure ulcer during his stay in the ICU. The case could not be considered without attention to the influence of the context: the ICU.

TYPES OF CASE STUDIES

Case studies can be exploratory, explanatory, or descriptive (Yin, 2009). Description in a case study is the attempt to answer the who, what, where, when, and how questions. Explanation is the attempt to answer the "why" question. Prediction in case study research includes forecasting near-term and/or long-term behaviors or events (Woodside, 2010). Any of the three types of case studies can use single or multiple cases. Single cases are used to characterize a unique or rare case. Single-case studies are also ideal for situations in which an observer may have access to a phenomenon that was previously inaccessible. These studies can be holistic or embedded. An embedded case involves more than one unit of analysis in the same case study. Multiple-case studies are repetitive; that is, each individual case study is unique and could stand alone as a single case, but together they are a more powerful representation of the whole, as, for example, in the Kitson et al. (2008) study of the process of facilitation to support quality-improvement efforts.

Exploratory case studies are used to explore those situations in which the intervention being evaluated has no clear, single set of outcomes (Yin, 2009). Often exploratory case studies are undertaken prior to beginning primary or discovery research to develop hypotheses. Flugman, Perin, and Speigel (2003), for example, documented reports of increasing numbers of adolescents taking adult-education courses, determined the characteristics of these youth in comparison with those of older students, and investigated additional issues and questions, such as characteristics of adult-education programs serving youth.

Explanatory case studies describe suspected relationships that are too complex for survey research, and attempt to link program implementation with program effects. This type of case study looks for relationships among variables or causes for specific outcomes. For example, using a case study approach, Horrigan, Rocchiccioli, and Trimm (2012) explained the relationships among chronic kidney disease, renal pathology, and renal fatigue in a 33-year-old woman on dialysis.

Descriptive case studies provide a detailed profile of a subject, an intervention, or phenomenon within a real-life context. A classic example is the case report study of five homosexual males who developed a rare pneumonia. This case study led to the subsequent discovery of AIDS/HIV. The initial cases were a cluster of injection-drug users and gay men with no known cause of impaired immunity who exhibited symptoms of *Pneumocystis carinii* pneumonia, a rare opportunistic infection known to occur in people with compromised immune systems (Friedman, 1981; Hymes et al., 1981).

COMPONENTS OF A CASE STUDY

Yin (1994, p. 20) identified five components of research design that are important for case studies:

- A study's questions
- Its propositions, if any
- Its unit(s) of analysis
- The logic linking the data to the propositions
- The criteria for interpreting the findings

Case study *questions* are phrased as "how" or "why" questions. For example, Lo (2002) wanted to know how nursing students coped with stress over the course of a 3-year nursing program.

The study's *propositions* focus the aims of the study and identify what data to collect. Propositions are derived from theories, literature, experience, or empirical data, and provide a framework for the case study. An exploratory case study, however, may not have propositions; rather, it will have a stated purpose or hunch as it seeks to explore a phenomenon as a prelude to primary research. The more a study contains specific propositions, the more it will stay within aims and time frame.

Examples of propositions from the research literature are:

- **Proposition**: Some women may choose not to have reconstructive surgery following mastectomy due to a fear of pain.

Source: Wallace, M. S., Wallace, A. M., Lee, J., & Dobke, M. K. (1996). Pain after breast surgery: A survey of 282 women. *Pain, 66*(2–3), 195–205.

- **Proposition**: For hospitals in which the elective surgery caseload is limited by nursing recruitment, to increase one surgeon's operating-room time, either another surgeon's time must be decreased, nurses need to be paid a premium for working longer hours, or higher-priced "traveling" nurses can be contracted.

Source: Dexter, F., Blake, J., Penning, D. H., & Lubarsky, D. (2002). Calculating a potential increase in hospital margin for elective surgery by changing operating room time allocations or increasing nursing staffing to permit completion of more cases: A case study. *Anesthesia and Analgesia, 94*(1), 138–142.

The *unit of analysis* is a critical factor in case study research. To determine the specific unit of analysis in a case study, ask the following questions:

- Do I want to understand something about individuals?
- Do I want to evaluate a program?
- Do I want to understand a process?
- Do I want to compare differences between groups or organizations?

According to Flyvbjerg (2011), if you choose to do a case study, the choice is less about what method to use, but more a choice of what is to be studied. The individual unit may be studied in a number of ways; for instance, qualitatively or quantitatively, analytically, or hermeneutically, or by mixed methods. There may be more than one unit of analysis in a case study. For example, if the researcher decides to analyze student performance based on a new curriculum, the student is the unit of analysis. However, the researcher might also want to explore how the teacher taught the class and the classroom environment. In this case, the unit of analysis is actually the group, the teacher, and the classroom environment.

Linking the data to *propositions* and the *criteria for interpreting* the findings are the least developed aspects in case studies (Yin, 1994). The challenge is to reduce the volume of data collected within the context of the propositions and framework developed for the study. Pattern matching offers some solution. This technique compares an empirically derived pattern with a predicted one. If the patterns match, the internal reliability of the study is enhanced. Explanation building is considered a form of pattern matching in which the analysis of the case study is carried out by building an explanation of the case. This implies that it is most useful in explanatory case studies, but it is possible to use explanation building for exploratory cases as well as in a hypothesis-generating process. Explanation building is an iterative process that begins with a theoretical statement, then refines it, revises the proposition, and repeats this process continually until no further explanation can be determined (Tellis, 1997a, 1997b).

DEALING WITH VALIDITY AND RELIABILITY

Validity and reliability need special attention in case study research. Construct validity is problematic in case study research due to the high potential of investigator subjectivity. Yin (1994, 2009) proposed three remedies to counteract this: using multiple sources of evidence, establishing a chain of evidence, and having a draft case study report reviewed by key informants (member checking).

Internal validity is a concern only in explanatory cases. This is usually a problem of interpretation in case studies, and can be dealt with using pattern matching, described previously.

External validity deals with knowing whether the results are generalizable beyond the immediate case; the more variations in places, people, and procedures a case study can withstand and still yield the same findings, the more external validity. An exacting literature review helps ensure external validity.

Reliability refers to the stability, accuracy, and precision of measurement. Reliability is achieved in many ways in a case study. One of the most important methods is the development of the case study protocol. A case study protocol contains the procedures and general rules that will be followed when constructing the case. A typical protocol should have the following sections:

- An overview of the case study project (objectives, issues, and rationale for a case study approach; topics being investigated)
- Field procedures (how permission will be obtained to access sites for data collection; what sources of information will be sought)

- Case study questions (specific questions that guide data collection)
- An outline for the final case report (Yin, 1994, p. 64)

COLLECTING CASE STUDY DATA

There are six primary sources of evidence used in case study research (Table 4.2):

1. Documents
2. Archival records
3. Interviews (open ended or focused; surveys are also used)
4. Direct observations (formal or casual)
5. Participant observation
6. Physical artifacts

Not all sources of data are necessary for every case study. Each case will require a unique set of data to be collected. Documents could be letters, memoranda, agendas, meeting minutes, policies, procedures, newspaper articles, or any document relevant to the case. The documents serve to corroborate the evidence from other sources. Documents are also useful for making inferences about events. Documents are communications between parties in the study.

Archival documents can be service records, organizational records, organizational charts, lists of names, survey data, maps, and other such records. The investigator has to be careful in evaluating the accuracy of the records before using them. Even if the records are quantitative, they might still not be accurate.

Interviews are one of the most important sources of case study information. They can be either open ended or focused, structured or episodic. In an open-ended interview, key respondents are asked to comment about certain events. They may propose solutions or provide insight into events. They may also corroborate evidence obtained from other sources. It is necessary to interview more than one informant to avoid becoming dependent on a single source of information. The focused interview is used in a situation in which the respondent is interviewed for a short period of time, usually answering set questions. This technique is often used to confirm data collected from another source. The structured interview is similar to a survey, and is used to gather data in cases such as neighborhood studies. The questions are detailed and developed in advance, much as they are in a survey.

Direct observation occurs when a field visit is conducted during the case study. It could be as simple as casual data-collection activities or formal protocols to measure and record behaviors. This technique is useful for providing additional information about the topic being studied. Authenticity of collected data is enhanced when more than one observer is used. Observation provides access to what people actually do in a situation, rather than what they have written or explained. In conducting an observation, watching what people do and listening

TABLE 4.2 Types of Evidence

Source of Evidence	Strengths	Weaknesses
Documentation	Exact names and dates of events provided	May be difficult to find or unavailable
	Exist prior to the case study	May reflect the bias of the author
	Can be used to corroborate evidence collected from other sources	Inaccurate or incomplete information may be contained in the document
Archival records	Can provide multiple levels of evidence (individual, community)	May be difficult to find or unavailable
	Can provide a detailed description of events over time	Health Insurance Portability and Accountability Act rules might inhibit some access
Interviews	Can be focused on the case study	Unskilled interviewer
		Poorly written questions
		Poor recollection
		Reflexivity may be present, i.e., the interviewee expresses what interviewer wants to hear
Direct observation	Reveals reality in real time	Time-consuming
		Observer may change dynamics
Participant observation	Provides insight into personal behavior	May be biased by investigator's subjective response
Physical artifacts	Offers insight into cultural features	May be unavailable
	Provides insight into technical operations	

Adapted from Yin (1994, p. 80).

to what people say is detached observation. For example, if the case study involves the elderly with communication or mobility difficulties, then observation is going to be more productive than interviews (Gillham, 2010). Participant observation makes the researcher into an active participant in the events being studied. This often occurs in studies of neighborhoods or groups. The technique provides some unusual opportunities for collecting data, but could present some major problems as well. The researcher could well alter the course of events as part of the group, which may not be helpful to the study.

Physical artifacts can be tools, instruments, samples of student's work, journals, or some other physical evidence that may be collected during the study as part of a field visit. The perspective of the researcher can be broadened as a result of the discovery.

ANALYZING CASE STUDY EVIDENCE

Analyzing results for a case study tends to be opinion based rather than based on a statistical method. The primary idea is to collate the data into a manageable form and to construct a narrative around it. Miles and Huberman (1994) suggested analytic techniques such as rearranging the arrays, i.e., the data selected for analysis; placing the evidence in a matrix of categories; creating flowcharts or data displays; tabulating the frequency of different events; using means, variances, and cross-tabulations to examine the relationships among variables; and other such techniques to facilitate analysis. See Table 4.3 for suggestions how to make meaning from case study data.

There must first be an analytic strategy that will lead to conclusions. Yin (1994) presented two strategies for general use: rely on theoretical propositions of the study and then analyze the evidence based on those propositions.

Pattern matching is another major mode of analysis. This type of logic compares an empirical pattern with a predicted one.

Yin (1994) encouraged researchers to make every effort to produce an analysis of the highest quality. In order to accomplish this, he presented four important principles:

- Show that the analysis relied on all the relevant evidence
- Include all major rival interpretations in the analysis
- Address the most significant aspect of the case study
- Use the researcher's prior expert knowledge to further the analysis

TABLE 4.3   Strategies for Making Meaning From a Case Study

What Goes With What
Noting patterns
Clustering
Seeing plausibility

What's There
Making metaphors
Counting

Sharpen Our Understanding
Making comparisons
Partitioning variables

See Things and Their Relationships More Abstractly
Subsuming particulars into the general
Factoring
Noting relations between variables
Finding intervening variables

Assemble a Coherent Understanding of the Data
Building a logical chain of evidence
Making conceptual/theoretical coherence

Adapted from Miles and Huberman (1994).

THE PROCESS OF CASE STUDY INQUIRY

Stake (1995) and Yin (1994) have provided guidelines for the development of a case study, including:

1. *Form a question and determine the objectives for the case study.*

As with all research, case study research begins with the formulation of a question and, with case studies, the setting of boundaries. For example, statistical analysis may have shown that maternal and infant mortality in some African countries is increasing. A case study can be a powerful and focused tool for determining the social and economic pressures driving this. However, can the researcher study both infant and maternal mortality in a reasonable time frame? And what country(ies) would be the focus?

2. *Conduct a review of the literature.*

To assist in framing the question, researchers conduct a literature review. This review establishes what research has been previously conducted and leads to refined, insightful questions about the problem (Zucker, 2001). A precise question can identify the keywords to use in the literature search, the methods of data collection, and the method of analysis to be used in the study.

3. *Develop a plan.*

A plan is necessary so that all relevant and important information can be obtained. Ask the following questions:

- What method of case study inquiry will best answer my question?
- What stakeholders need to be involved and/or interviewed or surveyed?
- What information is needed, where/how can it be obtained, and how will it be analyzed? See Table 4.4 for an example.

TABLE 4.4   Case Study Data Plan

Focus	Data-Collection Method	Data Analysis Method
1. Describe organization-wide policies and procedures related to the use of documentation	Documentation review	Content analysis
2. Usefulness of training sessions for nursing staff	Program evaluation	Statistical analysis
3. Nurses' attitudes, satisfaction, and perceptions of safety and quality regarding electronic documentation: before implementation	Questionnaire	Statistical analysis One-way analysis of variance
4. Nurses' attitudes, satisfaction, and perceptions of safety and quality regarding electronic documentation: 3 months after implementation	Questionnaire	Statistical analysis *T*-test
5. Nurses' ease of use and knowledge regarding computers	Questionnaire	Statistical analysis One-way analysis of variance
6. Change in workflow patterns, including documentation at the point of care	Interview Observation Time-and-motion study	Content analysis Statistical analysis: descriptive
7. Consistency/completeness of nursing documentation	Chart review Electronic health record review	Content analysis
8. Communication	Review of meeting minutes, memos	Content analysis

Source: Estrada (2008). (See exemplar at end of chapter.)

4. *Find and/or develop instruments for data collection.*

The rules or procedures that guide the collection of data are an important part of case study inquiry. This requires attention to development of an informed consent for those who will be interviewed or surveyed. As well, it is important to:

- Develop an interview schedule for each stakeholder or stakeholder group that lists the questions or issues to be explored that are relevant to that group
- Find, adapt, or develop a survey tool for each stakeholder or stakeholder group that lists the questions or issues to be explored that are relevant to that group

5. *Train data collectors.*

Find and train data collectors, if appropriate. Training should include: the objectives of the study, a review of data-collection methods, practice in the use of data-collection tools (including role play for interviews), the importance of confidentiality. It is also important to delineate the methods of record keeping with which trainers must comply.

Finally, a dissemination plan needs to be developed that outlines how the results of the case study will be shared and to whom they will be presented.

REPORTING THE CASE STUDY

Case studies frequently contain a strong element of narrative about the sequence of events and their relationship to each other and to context (Flyvbjerg, 2011). The researcher should use examples in the narrative while keeping things concise and interesting. It is useful to show some numerical data but remember that you are only trying to judge trends and not analyze every last piece of data. Constantly refer back to your bullet points so that you do not lose focus. It is always a good idea to assume that the person reading your research may not possess a lot of knowledge of the subject, so write accordingly.

In addition, unlike a scientific study that deals with facts, a case study is based on opinion and is very much designed to provoke reasoned debate. There really is no right or wrong answer in a case study.

The use of narrative involves a danger, however, of committing what has been called the narrative fallacy (Flyvbjerg, 2011). This fallacy consists of a human propensity to simplify data through a predilection for compact stories over complex data sets. It is easier for the human mind to remember and make decisions on the basis of stories with meaning than to remember strings of data. This is one reason why narrative case studies are so powerful and why many of the classics in case study research are written in the narrative format. But humans read meaning into data and compose stories, even when this is unwarranted. In case study research, the way to avoid the narrative fallacy is no different from the way to avoid other error; that is, the usual consistent checks for validity and reliability in how data are collected, analyzed, and presented.

Writing a case study research report is a challenge due to the variety of different kinds of evidence gathered in different ways, the skill required in weaving this evidence into a coherent narrative, and the need to maintain the focus and direction determined by the overall aims and the specific research questions. Exemplary case studies report the data in a way that transforms a complex issue into one that can be understood, allowing the reader to question and examine the study and reach an understanding independent of the researcher. The goal of the written report is to portray a complex problem in a way that conveys a vicarious experience to the reader (Zucker, 2010). See Table 4.5 for an outline for a case study report.

TABLE 4.5 Suggested Outline for Presenting Case Studies

1. The problem
    i. Identify the problem.
    ii. Explain why the problem is important.
    iii. How was the problem identified?
    iv. Was the process for identifying the problem effective?
2. Steps taken to address the problem
3. Results
4. Challenges and how they were met
5. Beyond results
6. Lessons learned

CONCLUSION

Case studies are complex because they generally involve multiple sources of data, may include multiple cases within a study, and produce large amounts of data for analysis. Researchers from many disciplines use the case study method to build on theory, to produce new theory, to dispute or challenge theory, to explain a situation, to provide a basis to apply solutions to situations, and to explore or describe an object or phenomenon. The advantages of the case study method are its applicability to real life; contemporary, human situations; and its public accessibility through written reports. Case study results relate directly to the everyday experience and facilitate an understanding of complex real-life situations. When using this method, enough detail must be provided so that readers can assess validity or credibility. To achieve this: (a) there must be a clearly written research question that guides the study; (b) the type of case study design chosen must be appropriate for the research question; (c) purposeful sampling strategies have been used; (d) data-collection strategies must be transparent; (e) the appropriate analytic method is used; and (f) the phenomena are viewed and explored from multiple perspectives (triangulation) (Baxter & Jack, 2008).

The goal of the case study method is to provide the most accurate description possible given the available data. Miles and Huberman (1994) have described 13 strategies for generating meaning from qualitative data. Such tactics range from descriptive to explanatory and from concrete to abstract (see Table 4.3). According to Miles and Huberman, the first three tactics tell us "what goes with what." The next two tell us "what's there," the next two help "sharpen our understanding." The next four help us "see things and their relationships more abstractly." Finally, the last two help us to "assemble a coherent understanding of the data" (pp. 245–246).

REFLECTIVE EXERCISES

Identify a topic that you would like to study; for example, "How is the process of nurses' bedside report going?" Answer the following questions:

1. Why would this be a case study?
2. What case study approach would work best?
3. What is the unit of analysis?
4. What are one or two propositions underlying the question? What is the source of the propositions?
5. What data would I need to collect to answer the question?
6. What will I do with the findings of the study?

REFERENCES

Baxter, P., & Jack, S. (2008). Qualitative case study methodology: Study design and implementation for novice researchers. *Qualitative Report, 13*(4), 544–559. Retrieved from http://www.nova.edu/ssss/QR/QR13-4/baxter.pdf

Brandell, J., & Varkas, T. (2001). Narrative case studies. In B. A. Thyer (Ed.), *The handbook of social work research methods* (pp. 293–307). Thousand Oaks, CA: Sage.

Bromley, D. B. (1990). Academic contributions to psychological counselling: I. A philosophy of science for the study of individual cases. *Counselling Psychology Quarterly, 3*(3), 299–307.

Dexter, F., Blake, J., Penning, D. H., & Lubarsky, D. (2002). Calculating a potential increase in hospital margin for elective surgery by changing operating room time allocations or increasing nursing staffing to permit completion of more cases: A case study. *Anesthesia and Analgesia, 94*(1), 138–142.

Estrada, R. (2008). *A case study of the implementation of an electronic health record in preadmission units and day-surgery centers.* Unpublished manuscript. Newark, NJ: University of Medicine and Dentistry School of Nursing.

Flike, K. (2013). Pressure ulcer prevention in the intensive care unit: A case study. *Critical Care Nursing Quarterly, 36*(4), 415–420.

Flugman, B., Perrin, D., & Speigel, S. (2003). *An exploratory case study of 16–20 year old students in adult education programs.* New York, NY: Center for Advanced Study in Education, City University of New York. Retrieved from http://web.gc.cuny.edu/dept/case/adult_ed/Adult_Ed_TimesRoman_Final_Rpt.pdf

Flyvbjerg, B. (2011). Case study. In N. K. Denzin & S. L. Yvonna (Eds.), *The Sage handbook of qualitative research* (4th ed., pp. 311–313). Thousand Oaks, CA: Sage.

Friedman-Kien, A. E. (1981, October). Disseminated Kaposi's sarcoma syndrome in young homosexual men. *Journal of the American Academy of Dermatology, 5*(4), 468–471. doi:10.1016/S0190-9622(81)80010-2. PMID 7287964.

Gillham, B. (2010). *Case study research methods.* London, England: Continuum International Publishing.

Horigan, A., & Trimm, D. (2012). Dialysis and fatigue: Implications for nurses—A case study analysis. *Medsurg Nursing, 21*(3), 158–175.

Horrigan, D., Rocchiccioli, J., & Trimm, D. (2012). Dialysis and fatigue: Implications for nurses - A case study analysis. *Medsurg Nursing, 21*(3), 158–175.

Hymes, K. B., Cheung, T., Greene, J. B., Prose, N. S., Marcus, A., Ballard, H., . . . Laubenstein, L. J. (1981). Kaposi's sarcoma in homosexual men—A report of eight cases. *Lancet, 2*(8247), 598–600. doi:10.1016/S0140-6736(81)92740-9. PMID 6116083.

Kitson, A., Rycroft-Malone, J., Harvey, G., McCormack, B., Seers, K., & Titchen, A. (2008). Evaluating the successful implementation of evidence into practice using the PARiHS framework: Theoretical and practical challenges. *Implementation Science, 3*(1), 1–12.

Lo, R. (2002). A longitudinal study of perceived level of stress, coping and self-esteem of undergraduate nursing students: An Australian case study. *Journal of Advanced Nursing, 39*(2), 119–126.

Miles, M., & Huberman, A. M. (1994). *Qualitative data analysis*. Thousand Oaks, CA: Sage.

Stake, R. E. (1995). *The art of case study research*. Thousand Oaks, CA: Sage.

Tellis, W. (1997a, July). Introduction to case study. *Qualitative Report, 3*(2). Retrieved from http://www.nova.edu/ssss/QR/QR3-2/tellis1.html

Tellis, W. (1997b, September). Application of case study methodology. *Qualitative Report, 3*(2). Retrieved from http://www.nova.edu/ssss/QR/QR3-3/tellis2.html

Woodside, A. (2010). Building theory from case study. In *Case study research: Theory, methods, practice* (p. 1). Bradford, England: Emerald Publishing Group.

Yin, R. (1993). *Applications of case study research*. Beverly Hills, CA: Sage.

Yin, R. (1994). *Case study research: Design and methods* (2nd ed.). Beverly Hills, CA: Sage.

Yin, R. (2009). *Case study research: Design and methods* (4th ed.). Beverly Hills, CA: Sage.

Zucker, D. M. (2001). Using case study methodology in nursing research. *Qualitative Report, 6*(2). Retrieved from http://www.nova.edu/ssss/QR/QR6-2/zucker.html

SUGGESTED READING

Aase, K., Laugaland, K. A., Dyrstad, D. N., & Storm, M. (2013). Quality and safety in transitional care of the elderly: The study protocol of a case study research design (phase 1). *BMJ Open, 3*(8). doi:pii: e003506. 10.1136/bmjopen-2013-003506.

Bradway, C., Bixby, M. B., Hirschman, K. B., McCauley, K., & Naylor, M.D. (2013). Case study: Transitional care for a patient with benign prostatic hyperplasia and recurrent urinary tract infections. *Urologic Nursing, 33*(4), 177–179, 200.

Chaboyer, W., McMurray, A., & Wallis, M. (2010). Bedside nursing handover: A case study. *International Journal of Nursing Practice, 16*(1), 27–34.

A Case Study of the Implementation of an Electronic Health Record in Preadmission Units and Day-Surgery Centers

ROSARIO P. ESTRADA

Background: The paradigm shift to a paperless health care record is a complex and expensive undertaking requiring staff/administrative/organizational resources, creativity, energy, and commitment. Yet it is a necessary venture as two presidential mandates require adoption of electronic health records (EHRs) by 2014 with appropriations of approximately $20 billion designated to accelerate the federal goal of more quickly moving the adoption and usage of EHRs.

Purpose: The purpose of this project was to construct a case study on the implementation of an EHR on a preadmission unit and day-surgery center.

Method: Descriptive case study. Following Yin's (1994) recommendation that specific questions guide the investigator during data collection, the research questions guiding the study were:

1. How is a technological innovation diffused on nursing units?
2. How does staff influence affect the success of the diffusion?
3. What are the facilitators and barriers to implementation of new technology?

Data were collected using document review, observation (time-and-motion study), stakeholder interview, and a survey of nurses' attitudes about the use of computers.

Findings: There were no statistically significant findings on the paired sample t-tests comparing pre- and postmean scores on the nurses' attitudes toward computers scale ($t = 1.938, p = .094$ [sig. 2-tailed]). However, comparing the pre- and postimplementation mean scores revealed that nurses had more negative attitudes postcomputerization as evidenced by a decreased mean attitude score from 2.53 to 1.78.

An interview provided more in-depth analysis to understand this finding. Overall, the nurses preferred the EHR to paper records but wanted the EHR to better support their nursing practice. Nurses stated that there was no current policy and procedure for the EHR but training guidelines were being used for teaching.

A content analysis of open-ended questions about perceived facilitators and barriers provided similar results. Perceived facilitators frequently encountered by nurses with the EHRs were easy to use, accessible, legible, saves time, allows continuity of care, offers improved quality of patient care. Perceived barriers and problems with the current EHRs were not enough time, frequent computer freezing, unfamiliarity/computer anxiety, privacy/HIPAA (Health Insurance Portability and Accountability Act) considerations, time-consuming, lack of eye contact.

A time-and-motion study was included as a collection method in the case study research to assess the amount of time nurses use for documentation. Initially, results showed that EHR documentation time was 2.5 minutes longer than the paper chart documentation time. It was expected that more time would be used for documenting electronically because of the added facility-defined features such as mandatory fields or improved regulatory compliance and enhancement of screens/forms to include evidence-based practice of nationally recognized instruments (i.e., Braden scale and pain assessment). There were variables such as interruptions, lack of computer skills, and inefficient time use, which affect nursing workflow. If the workflow process could be streamlined and inefficient time eliminated or reduced, the hospital could generate an annual cost savings of approximately $119,891.

Review of policy and procedure described the organization-wide policies related to the documentation unit on paper record and electronic record. During the interview, the nurses expressed that there was no policy and procedure for the EHR but guidelines were used for training and orientation of the new EHR system. They were unaware of the electronic policy.

Conclusion: Initially, there was some resistance from the staff due to the change from paper to electronic documentation and some technical difficulties to overcome, but with the training, support, and follow-up provided, the staff were able to recognize the value of the system. Considerations for users' needs and preferences and administrative support are essential to promote EHR adoption. Results of this case study will be valuable to streamline EHRs and improve/redesign nursing workflow as well as to develop effective implementation strategies in the diffusion of the EHR hospital-wide. It was evident that the design enhancements and implementation processes would be very important in fostering staff attitudes and improving workflow performance.

REFERENCES

Miles, M., & Huberman, A. M. (1994). *Qualitative data analysis*. Thousand Oaks, CA: Sage.

Yin, R. (1994). *Case study research: Design and methods* (2nd ed.). Beverly Hills, CA: Sage.

Qualitative Descriptive Research

OBJECTIVES

At the end of this chapter, you will be able to:
- Explain qualitative descriptive research
- Compare and contrast qualitative research with other types of qualitative methods
- Explain purposive sampling in relation to a qualitative descriptive study
- Plan and conduct a focus group

KEY CONCEPTS

- Qualitative descriptive research is the preferred method for direct descriptions.
- Qualitative descriptive research is based on naturalistic inquiry.
- Focus groups are typically used to collect data for qualitative descriptive study.
- Focus group moderators need to be skilled communicators.

Qualitative research investigates experiences, social processes, meaning, perceptions, cultures, and unfolding context. The qualitative researcher attempts to enter a person's world and to allow the person's words to lead to greater understanding (Munhall, 2007; Parse, 2001). Descriptive research, on the other hand, is typically associated with quantitative study, but in its basic format is a summary. Together these two types of studies combine to form the qualitative descriptive method, the goal of which is a "comprehensive summary of events in the everyday terms of those events" (Sandelowski, 2000, p. 335); in other words, a direct description of events using the terms provided by the subject. It is the preferred method when an uncomplicated description is desired. Specific questions that provide undeviating descriptions of the phenomenon of interest guide the study. The more common approach is to view a qualitative descriptive study as exploratory. Questions are very broad; for example, "What are the factors that influence health policy in low-income countries?" "What do patients think about electronic health records?" "What strategies work best to sustain quality-improvement efforts?" Getting an answer might involve interviews, observation, and/or reviewing documents.

Those engaging in qualitative descriptive study "stay close to their data and to the surface of words and events" (Sandelowski, 2000, p. 337). In other words, interpretations of the results are of "low inference" with findings presented as a digest of the facts. By providing information that is of low inference means that the researcher is only describing what he or she sees or has been told. For example, if the researcher describes the behavior of a chief nursing officer (CNO) as visionary, the researcher is inferring that the CNO is imaginative, creative, and bold. This is an interpretation of the CNO's behavior, rather than a description. In a qualitative descriptive study, the behaviors of the CNO would be described as they occurred.

The primary aim of a qualitative descriptive study is to provide an accurate description of an event and the importance a subject applies to the event. There is minimal theorizing as the qualitative descriptive researcher is interested in obtaining straight answers to questions (Sandelowski, 2000). For example, Carusone, Loeb, and Lohfeld (2006), in a study of what nursing home residents thought about pneumonia care provided in a nursing home, interviewed only those residents deemed capable of remembering and discussing care provided for a recent case of pneumonia. Other examples of potential qualitative descriptive study are:

- Use of portfolios for doctor of nursing (DNP) programs
- Nurses' opinions of electronic health records
- Student–teacher interaction in online classes

CHARACTERISTICS OF QUALITATIVE DESCRIPTIVE RESEARCH

Qualitative descriptive (QD) study differs from other qualitative methods in several ways. First, the aim of QD study is neither thick description (ethnography), theory development (grounded theory), nor interpretative meaning of an experience (phenomenology). Second, if an interview is conducted to collect data, the interview guide is more structured and questions are asked that relate specifically to the experience or event being investigated. Third, QD is the least theoretical of the qualitative approaches. It is a way of gaining a beginning understanding of an informant's views on a specific topic (Neergaard, Olesen, Jensen, & Sondergaard, 2009). This may make the analytical process somewhat subjective as descriptions will always depend on the researcher's perceptions and preferences (Sandelowski, 2000). Reflexivity is an important process used to avoid bias. Reflexivity involves reflecting on the ways in which one's own values, experiences, interests, and beliefs can bias the research (see Box 5.1). Finally, QD is less time-consuming than other qualitative methods.

The qualitative descriptive method is not bound by theoretical assumptions as other qualitative methodologies are, such as grounded theory in sociology, phenomenology in philosophy, or ethnography in anthropology. QD study is based in naturalistic inquiry, the study of something in its own unique environment. According to Erlander, Harris, Skipper, and Allen (1993), the problem statement in a naturalistic inquiry does not have to be a question or even an objective; rather, it is an "expression of a dilemma or a situation that needs to be addressed for the purposes of understanding" (p. 49). The focus is

---

Box 5.1

REFLEXIVITY IN QUALITATIVE DESCRIPTIVE STUDIES

Reflexivity involves reflecting on the ways in which your own values, experiences, interests, and beliefs can bias the research. To engage in reflection and decrease bias, the QD researcher must:

1. Carefully consider the interview conducted and how much influence the researcher may have had on the conversations. The researcher must be able to ensure that personal perceptions and assumptions did not sway the findings.
2. An assistant observes the researcher during focus group interviews, which assists in limiting bias and researcher influence.
3. Conduct an audit with the assistant to corroborate how she or he arrived at the findings (to increase the validity of findings).

about how people understand or think about events or experiences with a focus on "how" and "why" during the interview. The value of this approach is its ability to raise questions and provide a foundation for construction of hypotheses.

CONDUCTING A QUALITATIVE DESCRIPTIVE STUDY

Planning a QD study involves attention to sampling, data collection, and data analysis.

Sampling

Because the primary aim of a QD study is a straightforward representation of an event or experience, purposive sample is generally used. Purposive sampling seeks to find subjects who have some specific knowledge or expertise relevant to the topic, in other words they are rich in the information needed for the study. There are many approaches to purposive sampling; however, maximum variation sampling (MVS), a type of purposive sampling, allows for the greatest diversity among subjects. MVS does not seek representativeness through equal probabilities; rather, this type of sampling seeks to include those with wide ranges of extremes in opinions or experiences, which allow for a broader understanding of the topic of interest. The assumption is that if a researcher deliberately tries to interview a very diverse selection of people, their aggregate answers can be close to the whole population's, and can be as representative as a random sample (List, 2004). When using MVS, all the extremes in the population should be represented. For example, for a study on a nursing unit of how well a new protocol on the bedside report is working, it is beneficial to conduct interviews with those nurses who have:

- The most years of experience
- The fewest years of experience
- Indicated that bedside report is working well
- Never given bedside report
- Expressed a dislike for bedside report
- Have little to say about bedside report

Data Collection

Data collection in QD studies is directed toward discovering the who, what, and where of events or experiences. Data-collection methods typically involve the use of focus groups, document review, or observation of a specific event (Table 5.1). Focus groups are the most common.

TABLE 5.1   Methods of Data Collection

Method	Description	Advantages	Limitations
Focus group interview	Focus groups are interviews of groups of 6–10 participants. Each focus group session should last 1–2 hours.	Findings emerge from a group with a special interest or expertise in the topic. Findings can provide a foundation for further study or instrument development.	Subjects are not equally articulate. Transcripts may be extensive and difficulty to analyze. The small group size limits generalizability.
Observation	Observation is the researcher's attempt to note and record all behaviors of interest to an investigation.	Observations are recorded as they occur so that there is no loss of information. Observation overcomes the discrepancy between what people say they do and what they actually do.	The researcher may be seen as intrusive. Only current observations or behaviors can be identified. Sampled time frames (e.g., 3 minutes or 1 hour) may not correspond to real-life events.
Document review	A review of recorded information relevant to the investigation, such as reports, memos, meeting minutes, etc.	Can confirm information gathered during the interview or observation.	May not be accessible. Documents may be incomplete or poorly written.

Focus Groups

Focus groups are discussions around a predetermined set of questions that are related to a specific topic or event. A list of focus group questions, called an interview schedule, should be developed beforehand. See Table 5.2 for an example. Focus group sessions should be audiotaped. The researcher (called a moderator for a focus group) should have an assistant available to be sure that the recording device works properly and to assist in taking field notes and attending to the logistics of the focus group (e.g., room temperature, refreshments). The role of the moderator is to keep the conversation going and to reduce any unrelated conversations. The moderator should be friendly and greet each person in the focus group. One of the important functions of the moderator is to ensure that no one member of the group dominates, and that all group members have the opportunity to contribute to the session. A moderator needs to remain neutral; one who appears to be an expert on the subject will close important avenues of discussion. The moderator must have the ability to use participants' words and statements to introduce new topics and refer to what participants have said as a basis for moving to the next topic or question. See Table 5.3 for other necessary skills of a moderator. Some materials needed for a focus group session are:

Notepads and pencils

Recording device

Flip chart or easel paper

Focus group questions

List of participants

Markers

Masking tape

Name tags

Refreshments

Watch

The focus group should consist of 6 to 10 participants. Fewer than 6 participants tends to limit the conversation, and a group larger than 10 makes it difficult for the researcher to keep the discussion on track and to record nonverbal communication. A focus group should

TABLE 5.2   Sample Focus Group Questions

Study Question: What do school-aged children think about obesity?

Time Frame: 1 hour

Focus Group Question 1:
Let's begin by going around the room, one at a time. Please start by telling us your name and your favorite activities.

Focus Group Question 2:
What does the word "obesity" mean to you?

Possible probe:

- What does an obese person look like?

Focus Group Question 3:
How do you think people become obese or _____ (insert a word the children used to describe obesity)?

Possible probe:

- Can you give me an example?

Focus Group Question 4:
Do you know anyone who is obese?

Possible probe:

- (If so,) what caused this to happen?

Focus Group Question 5:
How do you think it feels to be obese?

Possible probe:

- Can you tell me more about that?

Focus Group Question 6:
Would anyone like to share anything else?

TABLE 5.3   Moderator Skills

Ability to communicate clearly

Ability to listen, not talk

Ability to avoid expressing personal views

Ability to maintain a low level of involvement

Ability to remember what was discussed

Box 5.2

ICE BREAKERS

Who knew?
>   Go around the room and ask everyone to tell the group some-
>   thing about him- or herself that no one in the room knows.

Sentence completion
>   These can be put on a flip chart or white board. Ask partici-
>   pants to complete the following sentences:
>   If I could throw caution to the wind, I would _____.
>   If I could be any person, alive or dead, it would be _____.
>   I laugh when _____.
>   I cry when _____.

Who am I?
>   Go around the group and ask each person to write his or
>   her name on a label along with a characteristic of him- or
>   herself that starts with the same letter as his or her name;
>   for example: Shy Sally, Dynamic Dennis.

---

last between 1 and 2 hours, which is enough time for 5 to 10 questions (see Table 5.2 for an example of focus group questions.) The actual amount of time depends on the sample. Children, for example, may only be able to participate for no more than an hour. Questions should include some introductory or ice-breaker questions that are asked first (see Box 5.2 for examples of ice-breaker type questions). The best focus group questions are open ended, and the researcher will need to have some probes ready to keep the conversation moving, which means that the facilitator needs to be very familiar with the questions to be asked. Probes can be detail oriented, such as "When did this event happen to you?"; elaborative, such as "Tell me more about that"; or clarifying, such as, "I'm not sure I understand what you mean by 'on-boarding' of new nurses. Can you explain?"

Questions should move from the general: "What do you think about . . .?" to the specific: "What can be done about that?" The questions should match the purpose of the study.

The setting in which the focus group takes place should be accessible, encourage conversation, and comfortably seat 10 to 12 people who can easily view each other. When the last question has been asked, the moderator should begin to end the focus group session by summarizing the discussion and asking participants if they wish to share anything else. This is also the time for the moderator to clarify anything that was unclear and to verify the accuracy of the information discussed. The analysis process should begin immediately following the focus group session by writing a summary of the session. The moderator and assistant should share perceptions of the process and compare field notes. The tapes should be transcribed as soon after the focus group discussion as possible.

Document Review

Documents are any preserved recordings that provide confirmation of information obtained from interviews and observations. A document review is the appraisal of textual information, which can include letters, newspaper articles, reports, memos, meeting minutes, and so on. For example, in a study of nurse retention, exit interviews of nurses who left the organization would be considered a document. In some cases, a segmental review is necessary as all of the document may not be relevant to the study. Information retrieved from documents needs to relate to the study purpose. This is called the recording unit. Documents that are vague or incomplete may need to be discarded due to serious doubts about the quality of the document.

Observation

Observation is the act of watching. If the researcher desires, for example, to investigate what goes on in the nurses' lounge, the researcher can sit in the lounge for a specified time and record observations. The researcher can see and hear what nurses are concerned about. Observation is a good source of information for studies involving infants or young children, the mentally ill, or incapacitated persons, particularly when the variables of interest are physical or behavioral. Observation is also an important method for determining reactions to new treatments or compliance with new protocols. For example, observing the behavior of a patient for 2 hours after ingestion of a new drug will allow the researcher to determine whether any unexpected reactions occurred as a result of the drug. As QD study is exploratory, extended periods of observation may be necessary, and the observer needs to be sure that nothing is missed during the observation. Questions to ask when constructing an observation include:

- How long should the observation last?
- How often should each participant be observed?

- When should the observation be done?
- How should observations be recorded?

Data Analysis

Content analysis is used for QD studies to construct codes and themes. It is used to determine the frequency of words in transcriptions, documents, or observations. Coding is the first step in content analysis and provides its foundation. An original quote is a code. Several similar codes comprise a theme or a single assertion about a topic that shows the relationship to the codes. This method provides a means of measuring the frequency and order of words, phrases, or sentences within a specific context (Burns, Grove, & Grey, 2013, p. 528; see Figure 5.1).

To perform a content analysis, the verbatim transcriptions of interviews, the recording units of the document review, and the observations made are coded, line by line. There are computer software programs that will code data (e.g., nVIVO), but some qualitative researchers will code their own data using colored highlighters or sticky notes. According to Krippendorff (2004), six questions must be addressed in every content analysis:

---

18   The pain was so excruciating that I thought my head would explode. I could not

19   think or move or respond in any way. The pain was tremendous. It was unforgettable.

20   I agree, I felt the same way when I had a stroke. The pain was one of the single most terrifying

21   experiences of my life. I thought the world was ending as I knew it. Sometimes, even now, when

22   I think back to that day, I can still feel the pain, even though people have told me I would forget

23   how bad it was. I have not forgotten.

Word count

Pain = 4

Forget/unforgettable/not forgotten = 3

Theme: Unforgettable pain

FIGURE 5.1   Code Passage From a Study on Perceptions of Pain

1. Which data are analyzed?
2. How are they defined?
3. What is the population from which they are drawn?
4. What is the context relative to the data analyzed?
5. What are the boundaries of the analysis?
6. What is the target of the inferences?

As themes are developed, the researcher assigns a working definition to each code. Thus, when going through the transcripts or other recorded results, the definition is continually being challenged. New codes may have to be developed if they do not fit into the definition of existing ones. This is a circular method of analysis as the researcher goes round and round among codes, themes, and definitions. This process is ongoing until saturation is reached, a state when no new codes or categories emerge and that coding anything else would only produce repetition of themes.

To enhance the validity of qualitative findings, the following strategies should be considered:

1. Triangulation, which is the cross-checking of information from different dimensions. For example, at the end of a focus group session, the moderator can summarize the discussion and ask the participants if the summary captured the essential elements of the session. As well, the moderator and the focus group assistant can compare field notes recorded during the session.

2. Longer or multiple observations that can provide a more accurate picture of the phenomenon of interest than just a short or single observation.

3. Member checking, which is the review of findings with a subgroup of those who were interviewed to verify accuracy.

4. Audit trail, which is the keeping of detailed and accurate records of everything the researcher did throughout the study.

WRITING THE QUALITATIVE RESEARCH REPORT

The qualitative research report follows the traditional standard for writing research reports: abstract, introduction, aims of the study, review of the literature, sample, data-collection methods, data-analysis methods, findings, discussion, and conclusion. However, as the report is a subjective method of research dealing primarily with words and descriptions, it is necessary to communicate as clearly as possible what was done; the details of the design; how data were collected, transcribed, and categorized; and how final themes or descriptions were generated. This allows the reader to judge the credibility of the findings. The main focus should be the data. Participants should be generously quoted to illustrate a category.

CONCLUSION

Qualitative descriptive research is a broad inquiry method that uses unstructured data-collection methods, such as focus groups, observations, or documents. A qualitative descriptive design is used when an uncomplicated description is desired that focuses on the details of what, where, when, and why of an event or experience.

REFLECTIVE EXERCISES

1. Choose a public place to sit for an hour, for example, the library, a train station, a shopping mall, a coffee shop. Observe the people you see. Write a description of what you saw. Do not try to interpret what you think those being observed were doing, just describe what you see using everyday language.
2. Reflect on the following list of potential qualitative descriptive studies. Select one and write a research question and list of focus group interview questions for the study.
   a. An evaluation of a nurse-managed clinic
   b. The role of psychiatric nurse practitioners in group sessions
   c. The leadership style of CNOs

REFERENCES

Burns, S., Grove, N., & Grey, J. (2013). *The practice of nursing research: Appraisal, synthesis, and generation of evidence* (7th ed.). Philadelphia, PA: Saunders (Elsevier).

Chan, S. C., Loeb, M., & Lohfeld, L. (2006). Pneumonia care and the nursing home: A qualitative descriptive study of resident and family member perspectives. *BMC Geriatrics, 6*(2).

Erlander, D., Harris, E., Skipper, B., & Allen, S. (1993). *Doing naturalistic inquiry: A guide to methods.* Thousand Oaks, CA: Sage.

Krippendorff, K. (2004). *Content analysis: An introduction to its methodology* (2nd ed.). Thousand Oaks, CA: Sage.

List, D. (2004). *Maximum variation sampling for surveys and consensus groups.* Adelaide, Australia: Audience Dialogue. Retrieved from www.audiencedia logue.org/maxvar.html

Munhall, P. (2007). *The landscape of qualitative research.* Sudbury, MA: Jones & Bartlett.

Parse, R. R. (2001). *Qualitative inquiry: The path of sciencing.* Philadelphia, PA: Jones & Bartlett.

Sandelowski, M. (2000). Whatever happened to qualitative description. *Nursing in Research and Health, 23,* 334–340.

SUGGESTED READING

Burnard, P. (2004). Writing a qualitative research report. *Accident and Emergency Nursing, 12,* 176–181.

Knott, A., & Kee, C. (2005). Nurses' beliefs about family presence during resuscitation. *Applied Nursing Research, 18,* 192–198.

Mauthner, N. S., & Doucet, A. (2011). Reflexive accounts and accounts of reflexivity in qualitative data analysis. *Sociology, 37*(3), 413–431.

Moss, V. A., Pitula, C., Campbell, J., & Halstead, L. (1997). The experience of terminating an abusive relationship from an Anglo and African American perspective: A qualitative descriptive study. *Issues in Mental Health Nursing, 18*(5), 433–454.

Neergaard, M. A., Olesen, F., Jensen, A. B., & Sondergaard, J. (2008). Palliative care for cancer patients in a primary health care setting: Bereaved relatives' experience, a qualitative group interview study. *Palliative Care, 7*(1).

Nurses' Perceptions of Nursing Handoffs at the Bedside

JOAN HARVEY

Background: The purpose of the bedside nursing report is to communicate critical information pertinent to patient care. Studies regarding nursing reports indicate that information is inconsistent among nurses. Despite attempts at creating standardized reporting sheets and implementing reporting methods to guide nurses, a lack of consistency remains, which can be a detriment to patient safety.

Aim: The purpose of this study was to examine nurses' perceptions of nursing handoffs conducted at the bedside report.

Method: The study used a qualitative descriptive design. Data were collected using observation and focus group interview.

Findings: Two themes emerged: (a) Despite being a mandated activity with an established procedure, nurses make the decision as to what patients to include in the bedside report, what information to pass to the next nurse, and where the bedside report will take place. Some of these decisions are based on the comfort levels of nurses, varying degrees of nursing knowledge, positive and negative experience with process, concerns with data confidentiality, and level of patient acuity, (b) The presence of nurse managers on the unit at the time of the shift report positively influences staff accountability for the bedside report procedure.

Conclusion: Nurses are the gatekeepers of all patient information. It is the nurse who ultimately decides what information will be transferred during the reporting process and when, by whom, and where the transfer of information will occur. Despite the bedside report being a mandated nursing action, nurses still decide whether or not to perform this task.

Clinical Interventional Studies

OBJECTIVES

At the end of this chapter, you will be able to:
- Identify the steps in a clinical interventional study
- Compare and contrast pre-experimental design, quasi-experimental design, and true experimental design
- Understand the basic statistical principles, concepts, and methods for analysis of clinical interventional data
- Design strategies to ensure fidelity of the intervention

KEY CONCEPTS

There are three basic interventional designs:
- Pre-experimental design
- Quasi-experimental design
- True experimental design

- A consent form is a necessity for anyone doing research with human subjects.

- Interventional research studies involve manipulation of the independent variable.

- Interventional studies build knowledge about what works and what does not work given specific conditions and subject characteristics.

- A clinical intervention is any deliberate physical, educational, or verbal action directed toward accomplishing a particular goal.

- Demonstrating the fidelity of an intervention is a key methodological requirement of any good intervention study.

Clinical interventional studies use the scientific method to build knowledge. Building clinical knowledge in nursing implies an understanding of the person—as an individual or as a member of a family. The focus of a clinical interventional study can also be a community or a group or a program. An intervention is a single act, a series of actions at either one point in time or over a period of time, or collaborative actions with other professionals (Burns & Grove, 2009). Forbes (2009) defines a clinical intervention as an explicit act, treatment, or technology (physical, psychological, or social) focused on a specific patient (or health care) problem or need. Any of the following can be an intervention: taking a blood pressure (a single act), caring for a severely injured patient in the emergency department (a series of actions at one point in time), implementing a protocol to decrease urinary tract infections (a series of actions over time), or designing a new nursing unit (collaborating with other professionals).

Although interprofessional ventures are increasing in frequency particularly when intervening in patient care, Forbes (2009) reminds us that nurses cannot defer total responsibility for nursing care to interprofessional teams. He states:

> There are many nursing practices that are not subsumed . . . (continence, symptom alleviation, tissue viability, etc.) and many other topics in which nurses are the main clinical care providers (e.g., self-care support, patient education, health promotion). (p. 558)

DeJong, Horn, Gassaway, Slavin, and Dijikers, (2004) note that nursing interventions must be completely described and fit within a theoretical or conceptual framework. Thus, clinical interventional research is guided by theory. According to Fleury and Sidani (2012): "Theory provides an understanding of the problem the intervention targets, the nature of the intervention, and the mechanisms underlying anticipated improvement in outcomes" (p. 11). Melnyk, Morrison-Beedy, and Moore (2012) have noted that framing interventions with a theory acknowledges the importance of how the concepts fit together to influence outcome: "Without a theory serving as (a) guide, choosing which constructs to investigate and manipulate would be like going on a wild goose chase" (p. 49).

The choice of the right theory to use to frame a clinical interventional study begins with identifying the problem, goal, or aspect of practice to be investigated, not selecting the theory because it is familiar or popular. Different theories are best suited to different targets, such as individuals, groups, and organizations (National Institutes of Health [NIH], 2013). For example, when implementing a smoking-cessation program, the Transtheoretical Model may be useful. When installing a new electronic health record system throughout a facility, Rogers's Diffusion of Innovation may be the best model to use. Organizational change theory may work well when trying to change practice patterns (NIH, 2013). See Table 6.1 for examples of theories used in clinical intervention studies.

TABLE 6.1 Examples of Interventional Studies Using a Theoretical Framework

Reference	Intervention	Theory Used
Meraviglia, M., Stuifbergen, A., Parsons, D., & Morgan, S. (2013). Health promotion for cancer survivors: Adaptation and implementation of an intervention. *Holistic Nursing Practice, 27*(3), 140–147.	The three-component intervention included (a) development of one-on-one participant–provider support relationships, (b) attendance at 6 weekly classes, and (c) follow-up support for 2 months to encourage use of health-promoting behaviors	Health promotion with chronic conditions
Navidian, A., & Bahari, F. (2013). Impact of mixed, hope and forgiveness-focused marital counselling on interpersonal cognitive distortions of couples filing for divorce. *Journal of Psychiatric and Mental Health Nursing.* 1–9. doi: 10.1111/jpm.12058	Counseling sessions	An integrated model of hope
Weatherspoon, D., & Wyatt, T. (2012). Testing computer-based simulation to enhance clinical judgment skills in senior nursing students. *Nursing Clinics of North America, 47*(4), 481–491.	Simulation	Kolb's Experiential Learning Theory
Hoffman, A. J., Brintnall, R. A., Brown, J. K., Eye, A. V., Jones, L. W., Alderink, G., ... Vanotteren, G.M. (2013). Too sick not to exercise: Using a 6-week, home-based exercise intervention for cancer-related fatigue self-management for postsurgical non-small cell lung cancer patients. *Cancer Nursing, 36*(3), 175–188.	Low-intensity walking and balance exercises in a virtual-reality environment with the Nintendo Wii Fit Plus	Symptom self-management
Paradis, V., Cossette, S., Smith, N., Heppell, S., & Guertin, M. C. (2010). The efficacy of a motivational nursing intervention based on the stages of change on self-care in heart failure patients. *Journal of Cardiovascular Nursing, 25*(2), 130–141.	Motivational interviewing	Theory of Heart Failure Self-Care

The relevance or significance of a theory to the target population and intervention needs to be considered. According to Fleury and Sidani (2011), when determining the relevance of a theory to an interventional study, an evaluation of the theory's underlying assumptions, empirical support for the theory's propositions, concept definitions, and construct validity are essential. Of further importance are the theory's explanatory and predictive ability regarding the intervention being investigated.

DESIGNING INTERVENTIONAL STUDIES

A study design is a blueprint. Good study designs: (a) answer the research question asked, (b) control for confounding variables, and (c) have a large enough sample to determine statistical significance (Melynk & Cole, 2011). There are three types of interventional research designs (see Table 6.2): pre-experimental designs, quasi-experimental designs, and experimental designs. Before any interventional study can begin, however, informed consent is necessary (see Table 6.3).

Pre-experiments are inexpensive and the simplest form of research. This design is used to determine whether a particular area of study is worthy of further investigation. Although pre-experimental designs follow basic experimental steps, they do not have a control group. A disadvantage of pre-experimental designs is that they are subject to numerous threats to validity, making it difficult to eliminate the possibility of competing explanations. Examples include the following.

One-Shot Case Study. In this type of study, subjects are presented with a treatment, such as the effect of simulation on knowledge attainment. The aim is to determine whether the treatment (simulation) had any effect on the outcome (knowledge); however, there is no comparison group and no baseline testing. Without a comparison group, it is impossible to determine whether the outcome (knowledge attainment) is any higher than it would have been without the treatment.

One Group Pretest/Posttest Study. In this type of study, pretest data are collected. For example, in the study of simulation on knowledge attainment, an exam could be given prior to the simulation and then again after the simulation, which can indicate a change in knowledge levels. It is still not possible, however, to be able to know whether the change is a result of the treatment (simulation).

Static-Group Comparison. This design compares the outcomes of two naturally occurring groups, such as two nursing units or two classrooms. The groups remain intact. One group receives the experimental treatment and the other does not. Both groups are then measured. The

TABLE 6.2   Types of Research Designs

Design	Focus	Elements	Learn More
Pre-experimental	Exploration	Little is known about the topic under investigation.	Wyatt, T., & Hauenstein, E. (2008). Pilot: An online asthma intervention for school-aged children. *Journal of School Nursing, 24*(3), 145–150.
			Design: one group pretest–posttest
Quasi-experimental	Description	Depicts a topic through data collected to answer a research question or test a hypothesis. Lacks randomization.	Muntlin, A., Carlsson, M., Safwenberg, U., & Gunningberg, L. (2011). Outcomes of a nurse-initiated intravenous analgesic protocol for abdominal pain in an emergency department: A quasi-experimental study. *International Journal of Nursing Studies, 48*(1), 13–23.
Experimental	Explanation	Independent variables are used to assign subjects to interventional and comparison groups. Manipulates at least one variable to test the effect on the outcome of interest.	Mathey, M., Vanneste, V., de Graaf, C., de Groot, L., & van Staveren, W. (2001). Health effect of improved meal ambiance in a Dutch nursing home: A 1-year intervention study. *Preventive Medicine, 32*(5), 416–423.

researcher then compares the two sets of measurements to see whether there is a difference. This design attempts to make up for the lack of a control group; however, lack of a pretest does not allow the researcher to determine whether the intervention made any difference.

TABLE 6.3   Elements of Informed Consent

Title of the study

Purpose of the study

Name of the researchers involved in the study

Affiliation

Procedures

Requirements of the subject

How information will be used

Potential benefit

Potential harm (risk of participating)

Statement on ability to withdraw without consequence

Signature of subject and witness

Date

Quasi-experimental designs have both an experimental and a comparison group; however, subjects are assigned, rather than randomized, to groups. A list of quasi-experimental studies follows.

Pretest/Posttest Nonequivalent Group. In this design, there is both a control group and an experimental group. This might be the method of choice for the simulation study. Students could be asked to participate in a one-semester simulation experience, where the simulation would take the place of some clinical hours, followed by measurement of knowledge. Knowledge would be measured prior to the simulation and again after the program. Those students who participated in the simulation would be the treatment group; those who did not would be the control group.

Time Series Designs. Time series designs refer to the pretesting and posttesting of one group of subjects at different intervals. The purpose is to determine the long-term effect of the intervention; therefore, the number of pre- and posttests can vary from one each to many. In the simulation study, for example, knowledge could be measured immediately after the intervention, at 3 months, at 6 months, and at 1 year to determine whether the knowledge was sustained. When there is an interruption between tests to assess the strength of the intervention over an extended time period, the posttest is referred to as follow-up and the design is called an interrupted time series.

Experimental design employs both an intervention group and a control group, and a means to measure the change that occurs in both groups. There is an attempt to control for confounding variables, or at least consider their impact on the outcome, while attempting to determine whether the treatment is what caused the change. The true experiment is often thought of as the only research method that can adequately measure cause and effect. Examples of this type of design follow.

Posttest Equivalent Groups Study. In this study design, there is both an experimental and a control group. Group assignment is done randomly. Posttests are given to each subject after the intervention to determine whether a difference between the two groups exists. There is no pretest measure.

Pretest/Posttest Equivalent Groups Study. This method is the most effective in demonstrating cause and effect but it is also the most difficult, most time-consuming, and most costly to perform. The pretest/posttest equivalent groups design provides for both a control group and an experimental group and adds a pretest. To apply this design to the simulation study, students would be selected randomly and then placed in either the intervention group or control group. The intervention (simulation) would be applied to one group and a control (usual method of teaching) would be applied to the other. It is important that the two groups be treated in a similar manner.

Prior to using any of these designs, the intervention or experiment must be planned and tested to the extent possible. Planning involves a determination regarding who will be involved in the intervention, including the need for any stakeholders (e.g., patients); whereas testing may require practice sessions or a pilot test. An intervention (also called a treatment) can be any of the following (Burns & Grove, 2009):

- A strategy
- A technique
- A program
- Training materials
- Methods of motivation
- Policy implementation

The way in which the intervention is to be administered should be guided by an intervention protocol. The protocol can be supplemented by an intervention manual and fact sheets. The manual should include a description of the topic, including its theoretical foundation, and a reference list. The activities to be conducted as a part of the intervention, any needed equipment, and the mode of delivery should be clearly described. Any necessary handouts should also be included with a timeline as to when they should be distributed. The manual can contain standards for the intervention in terms of dose (i.e., the frequency and duration of the intervention). Depending on the intervention, it may be necessary to provide a verbatim script. Strategies for reinforcing key ideas, troubleshooting, and actions for dealing with unhappy participants can also be included. The manual should also contain a list of names with contact information if any questions or concerns arise during the course of the intervention. The advantages to developing and using a manual are the greater consistency and precision possible when delivering the intervention, which enhances internal validity (Santacroce, Maccarelli, & Grey, 2004). The manual should also contain directions and forms for recording the number, frequency, and duration of all subject contacts as well as any deviations from the protocol (Fleury & Sidani, 2012).

Those who are administering the intervention should be formally trained and supervised prior to the start of the study. According to Santacroce et al. (2004): "The purpose of training and supervision is to mold, refine, and expand the skills of professionals who have experience with the study population or type of intervention. Training and supervision are achieved through manual review, didactic seminars, and experience" (p. 65). Attention to the training of those who are implementing the intervention is necessary to ensure that the intervention is conducted as planned, that is, that the intervention has fidelity. An intervention can be said to satisfy fidelity requirements if it can be shown that each of its components is delivered in a comparable manner to all participants and is true to the theory guiding the intervention and the research aims. Demonstrating the fidelity of an intervention is a key methodological requirement of any good intervention study (Dumas, Lynch, Laughlin, Smith, & Prinz, 2001).

VARIABLES AND HYPOTHESES

Every interventional study has at least two types of variables: independent and dependent. The independent variable (IV) can be manipulated. An independent variable causes a dependent variable to react. An example of an independent variable is noise level. Noises levels can be kept very low (a library whisper) or very high (a jackhammer), and the level of noise can be measured in decibels. Response to noise levels would be the dependent variable (DV), as the way someone would react to a certain level of noise can be related to the type and/or volume of the noise. The results of the study would depend on how the test subjects reacted to the noise. Measurements could include heart rate, respiratory rate, anxiety or anger level, or galvanic skin response. Any variable that can influence the outcome of a study but is not part of the study is called a confounding variable. For example, a loud clap of thunder that occurs during the noise-level study could interfere with the results, as its level of noise or timing cannot be controlled.

The hypothesis is directly related to the guiding theory but contains operationally defined variables in measurable form. A hypothesis is a single sentence that expresses the possible relationship between variables. The null hypothesis (H_0) is what is tested by statistics. Because the null is being tested, it is believed that if the null is not true, then some alternative to the null must be true. The alternative hypothesis (H_1) is also called the research hypothesis because it is really the aim of the investigation. To conclude that there is no difference between two groups means an acceptance of the null hypothesis. However, if statistical testing shows that the null is not true, then it is rejected and the alternative hypothesis is accepted; that is, there is a difference between the group means. For example:

H_0: Noise at 120 decibels (amplified rock music) will have no effect on heart rate.

H_1: Noise at 120 decibels (amplified rock music) will increase heart rate.

VALIDITY OF INTERVENTIONAL STUDIES

A valid study represents what it was intended to represent. There are two types of validity: (a) internal validity and (b) external validity. Internal validity refers to the ability to determine whether a causal relationship exists between one or more independent variables and one or more dependent variables. In other words, did the treatment really affect the outcome, either positively or negatively? There are eight major threats to internal validity:

History. History refers to any event outside of the research study that can change or effect a subject's performance. This threat can be controlled by randomization.

Maturation. Maturation refers to the usual physiological or psychological changes that take place as a result of aging. It can be controlled by subject matching so that all subjects mature equally. Randomization also helps to control this threat.

Testing. Testing refers to the use of the same test before and after the intervention. The chances that subjects will perform better the second time is a concern. Use of a control group can help with this threat.

Statistical regression. Statistical regression, or regression to the mean, refers to the tendency for subjects who score very high or very low to score more toward the mean on subsequent testing. This can be addressed by dropping the outliers from the analysis, that is, those who score very low or very high.

Instrumentation. This threat refers to a change in the measurement tool used in a study. Changes in scores may be related to the difference in tools rather than the independent variable. For instance, if a pretest is different from a posttest, the change in scores may be a result of the second test being easier or harder. This threat can be addressed by ensuring that alternative forms of testing are reliable and equivocal.

Selection. Selection refers to the manner in which subjects are selected to participate in a study and the manner in which they are assigned to groups. This threat can be addressed by randomizing subjects to study groups.

Experimenter bias. This bias can effect results that skew the study in the direction wanted. It can be controlled through blinding.

Mortality. Mortality, or subject dropout, is always a concern and can be controlled by subject matching.

External validity refers to the generalizability of a study. In other words, can we be sure that the results of our study population represent the entire population? There are four major threats to external validity:

Demand characteristics. Demand characterisitics involve inadvertently letting the subjects know the hypotheses under study. When asked a series of questions about work environments and burnout, for example, subjects may be cued to the hypothesis. When subjects become wise to anticipated results (a placebo effect), they may exhibit behaviors that they believe are expected of them. This threat can be controlled by blinding and the use of control groups.

Hawthorne effects. The act of watching a performance can cause a change in that performance, as those being watched may want to perform at a higher level to make a good impression. This can be controlled by using a control group.

Order effects. Order effects refer to the order in which interventions are administered. According to Cohen (1995):

> Performance on a series of tasks often depends on the order in which the tasks are assigned. Order effects can confound experiment results when different orders are systematically (and

inadvertently) associated with treatment and control conditions. A set of exam problems might be completed more quickly in one order than another, because one problem might prepare you for another but not vice versa. So if a control group of students is presented test problems in a "good" order and the treatment group gets the problems in a "bad" order, then a positive effect of treatment might be washed out by the effect of order; or, if the treatment group gets the "good" order, the effect of treatment (which could be zero) might appear larger than it is. (p. 4)

Treatment interaction effects. The term *interaction* refers to the fact that treatment can affect people differently depending on the subject's characteristics. Potential threats to external validity include the interaction between treatment and any of the following: selection, history, and testing.

SAMPLING: SELECTING SUBJECTS

Sampling refers to selecting subjects for the study. The sample comes from the population or the entire pool of possible subjects. In a classroom where the entire population is relatively small, testing all subjects may be simple. However, it is not possible to test an intervention on every new baby that is born or every person diagnosed with heart failure or all adults with dementia. In this case, a smaller group or sample of the target population is gathered and tested and then inferences are made that are representative of the population. For a sample to be representative it must resemble the entire population in as many ways as possible, but particularly with regard to the variables that are being studied or any known factors that might influence those variables (Burns & Grove, 2009). A study sample is found using either random (probability sampling) or nonrandom (nonprobability) methods. Probability or random sampling refers to the potential for any member of the population to be included in the study, making the sample representative of the population at large. Randomization means a chance allocation of subjects to one of the study groups. It characterizes a process of selection in which each person or entity in a study has an equal chance of being chosen for either the experimental (intervention) group or the control group. Random sampling can be simple, clustered, or stratified. Simple random sampling can be achieved by tossing a coin, throwing a die, pulling a name from a box that contains all potential subjects' names, or by using a list of random numbers. This type of sampling can lead to an uneven number of participants in each group. To avert imbalances, random samples can also be stratified when some variables are known to

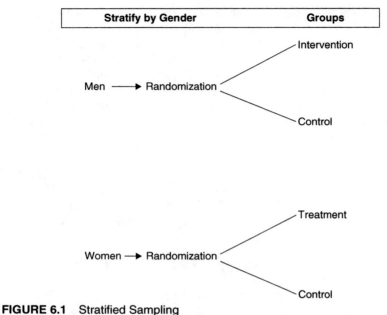

FIGURE 6.1   Stratified Sampling

be representative of the population, such as disease severity or gender (see Figure 6.1).

Cluster sampling assumes use of a naturally occurring group. Cluster sampling involves dividing the entire population (a state or a hospital) into clusters (zip code or nursing units), and then using techniques of simple random sampling within each cluster. The primary difference between cluster sampling and stratified sampling is that when using a cluster, the entire cluster is studied. When stratifying, a random sample is taken from within each strata. Data analysis is done by the cluster, for example, the results from the entire nursing unit; or by strata, for example, separate analyses for the men's group and the women's group. Cluster sampling can reduce the cost of the study; however, it is less precise than stratified sampling.

Nonprobability sampling does not involve a random selection of subjects. Rather, subjects are chosen based on their availability (or convenience) rather than their degree of representativeness of the population. Examples of nonprobability sampling include (Cochran, 2007):

- Convenience sampling, in which subjects are chosen based on their ease of access, such as a group of friends or students in one classroom.

- Snowball sampling, which involves a process of referral. One subject is selected, who then refers a friend, and the first friend refers a second, and so forth.

- Purposive sampling, which is based on the judgment of the researcher, who chooses the sample based on some predetermined characteristics.

- Quota sampling, which allows the researcher to choose any subject as long as a quota is met, for example, 60% of people in the study must be older than 50 years.

An interventional study can also be blinded. Blinding is to mask or hide something about the study or the intervention that might cause a bias in the study. For example, when testing the effectiveness of a drug on pain (vs. a placebo), the patient can be blinded as to what group he is in (intervention or control). This is known as single-blind testing. If a study were to be double blind, then both the patient and the researcher would be blind to group assignment. Random assignment of subjects to the experimental and control groups is a critical part of any double-blind research design. The identity of the subjects in each of the groups is kept secured by a third person. A triple-blind study is an extension of the double-blind design with the addition that the assessor is also blinded. The assessor is simply given data from patients who are in Group 1 or Group 2 (Holly, Salmond, & Saimbert, 2012).

The number of subjects needed in a study can be determined by a power analysis. This is a statistical procedure used to establish the number of subjects required to show a significant difference at the study's level of significance. There are two web-based programs that can help in determining an adequate sample size:

- *StatPages.net*. This site provides links to a number of online power calculators. It is available at statpages.org/#Power

- *G-Power*. This site provides a downloadable power analysis program. This program is available at www.psycho.uni-duesseldorf.de/abteilungen/aap/gpower3

ANALYZING RESULTS

A statistic is a numerical version of information ranging from simple computations such as determining the mean of a distribution, to the more complex determination of an effect size. There are two major types of statistics: descriptive statistics and inferential statistics.

Descriptive statistics use numbers to describe a known data set. For example, the average length of stay for patients with heart failure in the past 2 years would be a descriptive statistic, as we are using all of the patients with a diagnosis of heart failure during that time period. Inferential statistics are used to draw conclusions about a population and can be used for estimation or prediction; for example, the differences in test scores before and after use of simulated clinical laboratory activities. The specific statistical test used to analyze data depends on the type of the study and the level of data collected (see Tables 6.4 and 6.5); for example:

- Type of study:
  description (association)—correlations, factor analysis, path analysis
  explanation (prediction)—regression, logistic regression, discriminant analysis
  intervention (group differences)—*t*-test, ANOVA, MANOVA (multivariate analysis of variance), chi square
- Level of data
  nominal—chi square, logistic regression
  dichotomous—logistic regression
  ordinal—chi square
  interval/ratio—correlation

The results of statistical testing determine the significance of the findings. Significance refers to the level of confidence in the results of a study. In other words, if we want to be 95% confident in our results, we set the

TABLE 6.4   Levels of Measurement

Level	Characteristics	Examples
Ratio	Magnitude	Age
	Equal intervals	Height
	Absolute zero	Weight
		Percentage
Interval	Magnitude	Temperature
	Equal intervals	
Ordinal	Magnitude	Likert scale
Nominal	None	Names
		Lists

TABLE 6.5   Commonly Used Statistical Tests

Type of Data Analysis	Statistical Test to Use
Description	Mean, standard deviation
One-group comparison	*t*-test
Two-group comparison, unpaired	Unpaired *t*-test
Two-group comparison, paired	Paired *t*-test
Three-or-more-groups comparison, unmatched	ANOVA (one-way)
Three-or-more-groups comparison, matched	ANOVA (repeated measures)
Associations or relationships	Pearson correlation
Prediction	Regression

Note: ANOVA = analysis of variance.

significance level at .05 (or 5%). If we want to be 99% confident, our significance level is .01. If statistics estimate that there is 10% error and the study is set at a .05 level, the results of the study would be stated as "not significant." In this case, the null hypothesis would be accepted (Holly et al., 2012). See Box 6.1 for online resources to assist in data analysis.

WRITING THE RESEARCH REPORT

Research reports of quantitative findings from interventional studies follow a consistent pattern sectioned by the recommendations: Title Page, Abstract, Introduction, Methods, Results, Discussion, References, Appendices, and Author Note. The CONSORT statement, which stands for Consolidated Standards of Reporting Trials, provides a guideline for preparation of the final report (www.consort-statement.org).

Box 6.1

ONLINE RESOURCES FOR ANALYZING DATA

The Statistical Decision Tree
  www.microsiris.com/Statistical%20Decision%20Tree/how_
  many_variables.htm

Selecting Statistics
  www.socialresearchmethods.net/selstat/ssstart.htm

Interactive Statistical Tutorial
  statpages.org/javasta4.html#Demos

Title Page. The title page of a research report provides a brief summary of the report and should be no longer than 10 to 12 words.

Abstract. The abstract is the second page of the research report. It is a short, 200- to 300-word summary of the study, one paragraph in length, and contains no references. It follows the major headings of the research report.

Main Document. The main body of the paper has four sections: the introduction, which includes a review of the literature, methods, results, and discussion.

- **Introduction**. The purpose of the introduction is to introduce the reader to the topic and discuss the background of the issue at hand. The introduction also contains a review of the literature, which describes the current state of the topic that was investigated, plus the study objectives and hypotheses.

- **Methods**. The methods section is the second part, and refers to the procedures used to conduct the research. The study-design setting, sample, recruitment strategies, randomization methods, subject demographics, and pilot test results should be described in enough detail to allow transparency for replication.

- **Results**. The types of statistical tests used are described and results presented. Charts, tables, and graphs are often included. The results section should address whether the null hypothesis was accepted or rejected.

- **Discussion**. This section allows the researcher to describe the study, give its implications, and suggest areas for further research on the topic. Limitations of the study are also included here.

References. This section contains all the articles cited in the report.

Appendices. Appendices may be included at the end of the paper. Appendices should include only material that is relevant and that assists in understanding the study.

CONCLUSION

Because nursing is a practice discipline, an understanding of how particular interventions work and in what context they work best can inform the dilemmas of practice and improve patient care.

REFLECTIVE EXERCISES

1. Select a program that has been implemented where you work, such as a smoking-cessation program, an employee wellness program, or an AIDS prevention program. Determine:
   - The intervention specifications for the program
   - Key fidelity issues
   - Data used to determine the program's success
   - How human subjects were protected
2. The households in two areas of a large urban city are sampled to determine the level of physical activity of those living in the two areas. The areas are stratified into high-rent areas and low-rent areas. There are 100 households in the high-rent area and 900 in the low-rent area. Discuss the type of sampling that should be used for this study.

REFERENCES

Burns, N., & Grove, S. (2009). *The practice of nursing research* (6th ed.). Philadelphia, PA: Saunders/Elsevier.

Cochran, W. (2007). *Sampling techniques*. New York, NY: Wiley.

Cohen, P. (1995). *Order effects*. Retrieved from http://www.cs.colostate.edu/~howe/EMAI/ch3/node11.html

DeJong, G., Horn, S., Gassaway, J., Slavin, M., & Dijkers, M. (2004). Toward a taxonomy of rehabilitation interventions: Using an inductive approach to examine the "black box" of rehabilitation. *Archives of Physical Medicine and Rehabilitation, 85*(4), 678–686.

Dumas, J., Lynch, A., Laughlin, J., Smith, E., & Prinz, R. (2001). Promoting intervention fidelity: Conceptual issues, methods, and preliminary results from the Early Alliance prevention trial. *American Journal of Preventive Medicine, 20*(1, Suppl.), 38–47.

Fleury, J., & Sidani, S. (2012). Using theory to guide intervention research. In B. Melnyk & D. Morrison-Beedy (Eds.), *Intervention research: Designing, conducting, analyzing, funding* (pp. 11–36). New York, NY: Springer Publishing Company.

Forbes, A. (2009). Clinical intervention research in nursing. *International Journal of Nursing Studies, 46*, 557–568.

Holly, C., Salmond, S., & Saimbert, M. (2012). *Comprehensive systematic review for advanced nursing practice*. New York, NY: Springer Publishing Company.

Melynk, B., & Cole, R. (2011). Generating evidence through quantitative research. In B. Melnyk & E. Fineout-Overholt (Eds.), *Evidence-based practice in nursing and healthcare: A guide to best practice* (2nd ed., pp. 397–434). Philadelphia, PA: Wolters Kluwer/Lippincott Williams & Wilkins.

Melnyk, B., Morrison-Beedy, D., & Moore, S. (2012). The nuts and bolts of designing intervention studies. In B. Melnyk & D. Morrison-Beedy (Eds.), *Intervention research: Designing, conducting, analyzing, funding* (pp. 37–63). New York, NY: Springer Publishing Company.

National Institutes of Health. (2013). *E-Source: Behavioral and social science research*. Washington, DC: Author. Retrieved from http://www.esource research.org/tabid/36/Default.aspx

Santacroce, S., Maccarelli, L., & Grey, M. (2004). Intervention fidelity. *Nursing Research, 53*(1), 63–66.

SUGGESTED READING

Harkness, J., Lederer, S., & Wikler, D. (2001). Laying ethical foundations for clinical research. *Bulletin of the World Health Organization, 79*(4), 365–372.

Lopez, L. M., Tolley, E. E., Grimes, D. A., & Chen-Mok, M. (2009). Theory-based interventions for contraception. *Cochrane Database System Review,* CD007249.

Naylor, M. (2003). Nursing intervention research and quality of care: Influencing the future of healthcare. *Nursing Research, 52*(6), 380–385.

Whittemore, R., & Grey, M. (2002). The systematic development of nursing interventions. *Journal of Nursing Scholarship, 34*(2), 115–120.

Health Promotion in School-Aged Hispanic Children Through a Culturally Appropriate Nutrition and Exercise Family–School Program

MERCEDES ECHEVARRIA

Purpose/Objectives: The purpose of the project was to promote lifestyle changes for health related to diet and physical activity in Hispanic school children and their families. The specific objectives for this project were to:

1. Maintain or improve participant's preintervention clinical assessment findings.
2. Increase caregivers' knowledge of healthy nutrition and physical activity.
3. Analyze caregiver's dietary patterns based on national guidelines.
4. Promote development of consistent healthy patterns of nutrition and physical activity.

Hypotheses: (a) Participation in the educational program increases the caregivers' practices of healthy nutrition; (b) participation in the educational program increases the level of the caregivers' physical activity; and (c) participation in the educational program leads to reduction in weight for caregivers, improvement in body mass index (BMI) for school-age children, and improvement in blood pressure levels of both caregivers and children.

Methods: The research design was quantitative pretest–posttest using a demographic survey, the Health Promoting Lifestyle Profile II (HPLP II) tool, and pre- and postclinical assessments. A culturally and linguistically appropriate educational program was designed to promote family-oriented healthy nutrition and physical activity practices. Preliminary assessment of the neighborhood, school meals, and Hispanic family food and physical activity practices guided the development of the educational program. The windshield survey of the neighborhood surrounding the project setting was aimed to identify barriers to healthy nutrition and current levels of participation in physical activity by residents. The assessment included a review of neighborhood safety, parks and recreational facilities, transportation, and food establishments. Interviews with school lunch aides provided a preliminary assessment of students' food patterns and preferences. Recommendations for an improvement to the lunch experience included a less rushed atmosphere, maintaining proper temperature of food, offering ethnic foods, and finding creative ways to have children try fruits and vegetables. An interview with the director of food services provided an overview of federal mandates for school breakfasts and lunches. Children's free access to food, amount of time spent watching television, and participation in physical activity were addressed with caregivers during the parent–teacher meetings. The educational program designed for the project (the intervention) incorporated the findings of the preliminary assessment.

The program was implemented weekly for 10 weeks on consecutive Saturdays. The weekend schedule was chosen to accommodate the family-oriented participation in activities common among Hispanics. Each session consisted of 2.5 hours divided into two component parts: (a) 90 minutes on promoting healthy diet and lifestyle behaviors for the family and developing a family approach to incorporate traditional Hispanic food preferences into healthy cooking practices, and (b) 60 minutes of low-impact aerobic activity for the family. Areas of special interest to Hispanic families such as dancing and listening to popular Hispanic music were used. All learning activities were conducted in English and Spanish, which included lecture presentation, and fun activities such as a healthy food store tour, family health/nutrition bingo, and family physical activities.

Caregivers kept a daily log of their food intake and physical activity. Analysis of the weekly food and activity logs was given to each caregiver. Discussion of the analysis was done in a focus group format with individual counseling if needed. Findings were reported to participants as aggregate data. Pre- and posteducational program assessments were done using one instrument, the HPLP II, and clinical assessment of weight, BMI, and blood pressures.

Participants: Participants in the study were a convenience sample drawn from parents of school children attending one elementary school located in a predominantly Hispanic community. The sample comprised 14 caregivers and their school-aged children. The criteria for caregiver eligibility included: (a) self-identified as Hispanic, (b) having a child enrolled in the public school between preschool through fifth grade, (c) living in the same household as the child, (d) responsible for preparing or purchasing food for the child's household, (e) no self-reported medical condition that would prohibit physical activity, and (f) agreed to complete the 10-week project implementation period. Participation in this intervention presented no identified risks. An advanced practice nurse was available at all times throughout the intervention. A written consent form was offered. All participants were able to read and write. A written assent form was also offered to all children.

Findings: Hypotheses 1 and 2 were supported by paired-sample tests on the pre- and post means of caregivers on the HPLP nutrition and Physical Activity Subscales. With regard to Hypothesis 3, significant differences in the pre- and post-BMI and pre- and post-systolic blood pressure of school-aged children were found through the paired-samples t-test. In contrast, the t-test comparison on the caregivers was not significant. However, comparison of means in all parameters—weight, BMI, and diastolic and systolic blood pressure—revealed a change in the means from higher preintervention to lower postintervention. It is possible that because the sample was small and the mean differences were not pronounced, statistical significance was not achieved.

Conclusion: The study attempted to determine the outcomes of an educational intervention on knowledge and practices of healthy nutrition and physical activity in a group of Hispanic school-aged children and their caregivers. Implementation of a cultural and linguistic educational program is effective in changing nutritional and physical activity practices that can impact the health status of adults and children. The study demonstrated a successful model for recruiting and retaining Hispanic participants in a combined nutrition and physical activity intervention. The intervention was an important first step in designing an ongoing multidisciplinary nutrition and physical activity program and points to the need for continued research to decrease health disparities in Hispanics.

Project Limitation: Because of the project's time frame, evaluation of sustained outcomes over time was not possible. Because the study used a small convenience sample, the findings have limited generalization. All the participants were the caregivers and children who were recruited from one school. The project's focus was limited only to two areas of health promotion: nutrition and physical activity.

7

Systematic Review

OBJECTIVES

At the end of this chapter, you will be able to:
- Delineate the benefits of a systematic review
- Differentiate among the types of systematic review
- Outline the steps in a systematic review

KEY CONCEPTS

- A systematic review is a research method.
- Systematic reviews bring the same level of rigor to the research process found in primary studies.
- Systematic reviews may be conducted using quantitative evidence, qualitative evidence, or both.
- Systematic reviews provide a balanced and impartial summary of findings with consideration given to the strengths and weaknesses of included studies.
- The findings of a systematic review can provide the foundation for primary research.

A systematic review is a descriptive research method in which the subjects or informants in the study are published or unpublished primary studies rather than human subjects. The word *systematic* refers to a logical and orderly approach that mirrors the one used in primary studies. Systematic reviews are an accepted form of research, the findings of which allow practitioners to make point-of-care decisions based on the best available evidence for a focused clinical question. It is preferred practice to look at a body of evidence when making health care

TABLE 7.1   Benefits of a Systematic Review

A clear question guides the review

Collapses large amounts of information critically appraised to be rigorous into a manageable, usable format

Provides clearer and less biased understanding because of the systematic process and the checks and balances of two researchers

Increases the strength and generalizability/transferability of the findings because they are derived from a broader range of populations, settings, circumstances, treatment variations, and study designs

Minimizes bias from random and systematic error

Pools and synthesizes existing information for decisions about clinical care, economic decisions, future research design, and policy formation

Assesses consistencies and provides explanations for inconsistencies of relationships across studies

Increases power in suggesting cause-and-effect relationships

Increases confidence in conclusions

Increases likelihood of results being used in clinical practice

Provides a format for ongoing updates of new evidence

Helps practitioners keep up to date with overwhelming quantities of medical literature

Source: Holly, Salmond, and Saimbert (2012).

decisions, rather than the results of one study (Chalmers, 2006). The benefits of systematic review are many (Table 7.1) and include:

- Providing reliable evidential summaries of completed research that are more powerful than the results of a single study
- Providing outcome data that can be used in policy decisions
- Clarifying existing data to avoid duplication in research studies
- Helping practitioners stay current with overwhelming quantities of health-related literature

TYPES OF REVIEWS

There are two basic types of systematic review: a quantitative meta-analysis, which uses the results of randomized controlled trials or observational studies; and a qualitative meta-synthesis, which uses the results of phenomenology, grounded theory, ethnography, action research, or other qualitative methods. Meta-analysis and meta-synthesis are umbrella terms for the way in which data are analyzed within a systematic review.

Meta-Analysis

Meta-analysis is statistical synthesis of data that are pooled for analysis from a set of similar studies on the same topic. The general aim of a meta-analysis is to estimate the effect of interventions or treatments under a given single set of assumptions and conditions. It is a systematic investigation of effect sizes and the exploration of their variations across studies. For instance, a meta-analysis may be conducted using the results of several clinical trials of a drug treatment or a self-care management educational intervention in an effort to obtain a better understanding of how well the treatment or intervention worked. A summary of the pooled results, called an effect size, is provided. Studies used in a meta-analysis can be experimental or descriptive, although the preferred study for use is the randomized controlled trial (RCT). An RCT is a carefully controlled clinical trial that studies the effect of a therapy (intervention or treatment) on actual patients. Attention is paid to randomization to study group (experimental or control group), blinding, and bias.

Observational studies can also be used in a review. These include cohort studies, case-control studies, case series, or case reports. Cohort studies follow a large population over time. Subjects have the same condition (e.g., diabetes) or receive the same treatment over time (e.g., chemotherapy). Comparisons are made with another group without condition or treatment being studied. Case-control studies are about patients who already have a specific condition (e.g., HIV/AIDS). Patient outcomes are compared with those who do not have this condition. Medical records and patient historical recall are used to collect data. Case series and case reports are narratives about the treatment of individual or groups of patients; there are no controls or comparisons (Holly, Salmond, & Saimbert, 2012).

Meta-analysis is conducted using a predetermined model for analysis. A fixed-effect model provides a weighted average of the study estimates, in which the weights are the inverse variance of the study estimate. Consequently, studies with a larger sample size are given greater weight in the analysis regardless of the significance of findings. In other words, larger studies dominate the analysis. Smaller studies, though significant in their findings, can be ignored. Fixed-effect models are useful when there is certainty that the underlying effects are the same for all studies. As this is rarely the case in health-related research, findings may be difficult to interpret, including having a very narrow confidence interval. To allow for the differences between health-related studies (called heterogeneity), a random-effect model should be used. In this model, the weight of each study is redistributed, and an unweighted average for the effect size is determined across studies, equalizing the studies regardless of sample size (Box 7.1).

Box 7.1

HETEROGENEITY

Heterogeneity is about clinical variation. In health-related research this can be due, for example, to differences in the sample (age, gender, comorbidities), study site (hospital, nursing home, clinic, home care agency), or condition (severity of illness).

The chi-squared test provides an indication of the significance for heterogeneity, but it does not measure it. A measurement index for heterogeneity is provided by the I_2, a percentage of the chi-squared statistic, which is not explained by the variation within the studies. It represents the percentage of the total variation due to variation between studies.

To interpret I_2:
$I_2 = \ \ 0\%$—no heterogeneity
$I_2 = 25\%$—low heterogeneity
$I_2 = 50\%$—moderate heterogeneity
$I_2 = 75\%$—high heterogeneity

In this example: $I_2 = 71\%$, $P = .003$, shows that there is a high level of heterogeneity and the chi-square result determines that this is a significantly high level. In this case, a determination has to be made as to whether there is too much variation to pool the studies or a narrative review should be conducted.

REFERENCES
Higgins, J. P. T., & Thompson, S. G. (2002). Quantifying heterogeneity in a meta-analysis. *Statistics in Medicine, 21*, 1539–1558.
Higgins, J. P. T., Thompson, S. G., Deeks, J. J., & Altman, D. G. (2003). Measuring inconsistency in meta-analyses. *British Medical Journal, 327*, 557–560.

A new model, called a quality model, is gaining popularity. In this model, study quality is used in combination with study weight. This allows the methodological quality of a study, determined during the appraisal process, to be used along with study findings when analyzing results. In other words, if one study is of good quality and other studies are of poor quality, a proportion of their quality-adjusted weights is mathematically redistributed, giving it more weight toward the overall effect size. As studies increase in quality, redistribution becomes progressively less necessary and ceases when all studies are of perfect quality (Doi & Thalib, 2008). A software program is available to conduct this analysis as a free add-on to Excel (MetaXL, 2012).

Meta-Synthesis

Meta-synthesis is a broad term that refers to the qualitative aggregation or interpretation of the findings from qualitative studies. Studies used in meta-synthesis include: (a) phenomenology, which presents the lived experiences and the meaning of that experience from the viewpoint of the subject, and aims to provide a greater depth of understanding about the experiences in people's lives; (b) grounded theory, which explores social processes among humans and generates new theoretical constructs that illuminate human behavior in a social world; (c) ethnography, which attempts to show how people in a specific culture or subculture make sense of their experiences and realities; (d) action research, which uses a specific process to improve a situation; or (e) qualitative descriptive studies, which provide an uncomplicated description of events using the words of interviewed subjects.

The findings drawn from these various methods are translated one into another using colloquial, rather than word-for-word, translation "creating a broader and deeper understanding of the phenomenon" under investigation (Holly et al., 2012, p. 224). Translating means that similar concepts are identified in each individual study, although they may be expressed differently. These concepts are combined in ways that go beyond the original. This is primarily done through meta-aggregation or meta-ethnography. Meta-aggregation is the summing or integration of the original findings, which allows a comprehensive summary of statements that can be used as best practices. In contrast, meta-ethnography allows the researcher to deduce new meaning, rather than reinterpret original meanings. Findings are not aggregated but analyzed to create new knowledge and conceptual models of understanding.

STEPS IN A SYSTEMATIC REVIEW

Similar to primary studies, systematic reviews follow a specific methodology (Table 7.2). Steps in the systematic review process include:

Step 1: Formulate a Focused Clinical Question

A focused question is one that is useful to practitioners, leads to a change in practice based on new evidence, or increases confidence in usual care (Kitchenham, 2004). Typically, review questions focus on interventions or therapy, etiology or causation, diagnosis, prognosis, economics, or meaning (Table 7.3). A review question about what intervention or therapy works or is most effective is best answered using randomized controlled

TABLE 7.2   Steps in a Meta-Analysis

1. Formulate a focused clinical question.
2. Determine keywords and phrases. Search the literature.
3. Select studies.
   - Critically appraise each study
   - Include unpublished studies to avoid publication bias
4. Determine summary measures for extraction.
   - Differences (discrete data)
   - Means (continuous data)
   - Use a data extraction tool to extract all data
5. Choose a model for analysis.
   - Fixed effect model

     This model provides a weighted average of the study estimates. The sample size within each study determines how much weight is given to the study, which allows larger studies to dominate regardless of findings. This model is used when the intent is to generalize only to the review population.
   - Random effects model

     This model uses the confidence interval (a measure of preciseness) to determine the weight each study is given. This model should be used when the intent is to generalize to a larger population.
6. Interpret results and draw conclusions.
   - The conclusions drawn from a meta-analysis can be used as best practice recommendations, if appropriate.

Adapted from Holly and Slyer (2013).

---

trials. Questions of etiology or causation assist in indentifying the likely causes of a condition. Diagnosis or diagnostic testing questions are concerned with how well a diagnostic test works, and questions of prognosis deal with how to estimate the patient's likely clinical course over time and what complications are likely to occur. Cost underlies economic questions. Questions of meaning concern the experiences, perceptions, feelings, and opinions of the study participant about a particular topic or experience.

Well-formulated questions use the PICO format:

P stands for population, patients, or phenomenon of interest.

I is used to describe the intervention or approach to be studied.

C is for comparison, or main alternatives to the intervention to be studied.

O stands for outcome.

TABLE 7.3   Examples of Systematic Review Questions

Type of Review	Question Example	Best Study to Use in a Review
Intervention or Therapy	What is the effect of telephone follow-up and counseling vs. no follow-up in 90-day readmission rates for heart failure?	RCT Cohort Case control Case series
Etiology, Screening, Risk/Harm	What are the risk factors for development of coronary artery disease in Asian Indians?	RCT Cohort Case control Case series
Diagnosis or Diagnostic Testing	What test works best for the diagnosis of tuberculosis?	Prospective, comparison to a gold standard
Prognosis or Prediction	Over the course of 2 years, what happens to patients diagnosed with a chronic disease?	Cohort study Case control Case series
Economics	What type of PICC line decreases cost and site infection in children on chemotherapy?	Cost-benefit Cost utilization Cost minimization
Meaning	What outcomes are most important to patients undergoing treatment for obesity?	Qualitative

An example of a therapy question for a systematic review using this mnemonic is "In teenage boys (P), how effective is a peer counseling program (I) in reducing smoking (O)?" The comparison would be teenage boys who are not enrolled in the peer counseling program.

Systematic review of qualitative studies use a modified version PICO in which the C and the O are combined to mean context: PICo. For example, "How do family members (P) who witness an out-of-hospital cardiac resuscitation by emergency personnel (I) perceive the experience in the first month of grieving?" (Holly et al., 2012, p. 16).

Taking time to craft the question will make searching for relevant studies for inclusion in the review easier as the inclusion criteria are clearly evident in the question.

Step 2: Find and Extract the Right Studies

Searching for the right studies for a systematic review is the equivalent of data collection in a primary study. The PICO question is used to determine the keywords used for searching. In the example above, "In teenage boys (P), how effective is a peer counseling program (I) in reducing smoking (O)?" the keywords are "teenage boys," "smoking" and "peer counseling." To broaden the search so that nothing is missed, alternative words or phrases should also be used, such as "adolescent boys," "smoking" reduction/smoking-cessation programs." A concept map is useful in identifying all of the keywords and their alternatives (Figure 7.1). Randomized controlled trials (or other studies of effect) should also be an inclusion criterion as this is an effectiveness review.

To conduct the search, select the databases to be used that best represent either the field of the study (e.g., nursing, social work, psychology) or other health-related databases. There is no set number of databases to search; however, the search should be as exhaustive as possible so that all relevant papers are found. Each database selected for searching has a short tutorial on how to use the database and how words are indexed. It is important to watch these before beginning the search as each database indexes differently. For example, the word "handwashing" may have been entered into a database as "handwashing," "hand washing," or "hand-washing." When searching for nursing studies, the following databases are useful places to start:

1. Academic Search Premier
2. MEDLINE/PubMed
3. CINAHL and pre-CINAHL
4. EMBASE
5. Web of Science
6. ClinicalTrials.gov

When conducting a systematic review, it is important to determine whether a review of the topic has already been done. A search of the Cochrane, Campbell, or Joanna Briggs Libraries of systematic reviews or other review sites (Box 7.2) will help determine this. In the event a review on the topic is found, it can be extended if the review is 3 to 5

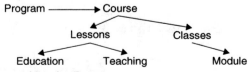

FIGURE 7.1   Concept Map for Program

Box 7.2

SYSTEMATIC REVIEW SITES

The Joanna Briggs Institute
 www.joannabriggs.edu.au

The Cochrane Library
 www.cochrane.org

The Campbell Collection
 www.campbellcollection.org

PubMed Clinical Inquiry: Find Systematic Reviews
 www.ncbi.nlm.nih.gov

Bandolier
 www.medicine.ox.ac.uk/bandolier

The NHS Center for Reviews and Dissemination
 www.york.ac.uk

---

or more years old. In this case, the review would need to be identified as an extension of the original work.

To decrease the bias associated with using only published studies in a systematic review, grey literature (unpublished) sites should also be searched. Searching the grey literature sites can provide conference proceedings, white papers, and other material useful to the review. These include:

- World Health Organization, Centers for Disease Control and Prevention, or state health departments
- *The Grey Literature Report*, a bimonthly publication of The New York Academy of Medicine Library
- National Technical Information Service (U.S.), the largest central resource for U.S.-government funded scientific-, technical-, engineering-, and business-related information available today.
- OAIster, a catalog of records representing open access resources, including theses, technical reports and research papers, and digital items.
- Google Scholar
- OpenGrey (formerly SIGLE), a bibliographical reference of grey literature produced in Europe.

- NLM Gateway (National Library of Medicine), which identifies studies and author contact information, particularly for clinical trials.
- The Virginia Henderson Library of Sigma Theta Tau International and Magnet Conference Proceedings provide abstract and author contact information.

Other methods of searching for relevant studies include hand searching, use of personal contacts (circle of friends), and reviewing reference lists (harvesting). Hand searching involves identifying journals that are directly related to the focus of the review (e.g., *Pain and Analgesia Journal* for a study on pain management). This is a time-consuming but necessary task as not all articles are indexed in electronic bibliographic databases. Personally contacting principal investigators of studies related to the review topic or other experts in the field can help identify unpublished or in-progress work. Each person contacted can be asked to identify other persons who might have additional information (snowballing technique). Examining the reference lists of simple reviews of the literature and those papers retrieved for the review can also help identify additional sources that can be added to the review (Holly et al., 2012; Littell, Corcoran, & Pillai, 2008).

For each database searched, a record should be kept that includes the date of the search, the title of the database (with URL address), the range of dates searched, and the results of the search (Littell et al., 2008). The assistance of a research librarian with knowledge of the process of systematic review would be an invaluable asset to a well-developed and well-documented search.

Step 3: Appraising Studies

When an exhaustive search has been completed, the studies retrieved for the review must be appraised for methodological quality. As the purpose of a systematic review is to establish whether or not the findings of primary research are consistent over time and over differing populations, the studies included in the review should be of the highest quality. A critical appraisal is done to determine the validity, value, and relevance to the particular clinical question under review. When appraising the validity of a study, attention to sources of potential bias, or threat, is essential. Threats include:

- Effects of repeated testing (pretest and posttest designs).
- Selection—Subjects who agree to participate in a study may be very different from those who refuse participation.

- Mortality/attrition—Subjects withdraw from the study before completion and may be very different from the subjects who complete the study.
- History—Events that occur during the conduct of the study may have influenced the treatment or the outcome. Therefore, the treatment may not yield the same results at a different time.
- Instrumentation—Use of the same test on multiple occasions may cue the subject to the hypothesis.
- Performance—The fact that a subject is in a research study may result in behaviors that are not usual.

There are several highly regarded tools that can be used for such an appraisal, such as CASP (Critical Appraisal Skills Programme; www.sph.nhs.uk/what-we-do/public-health-workforce/resources/critical-appraisals-skills-programme), and Joanna Briggs Institute tools (joannabriggsinstitute. edu.au). There are different checklist tools with questions for appraisal specific to the type of study being considered, such as RCT, cohort, or case series or meaning. The checklists developed by the Joanna Briggs Institute include one for appraisal of economic studies.

To begin the appraisal, the basic questions to ask regarding any research study are:

- Has the research been conducted in such a way as to minimize bias? If so, what does the study show?
- What do the results mean for the particular patient or context in which a decision is being made (Burls, 2009)?

Questions for appraisal then become more specific and focus on:

1. The clarity of the clinical question with regard to the population, intervention, and outcome (or phenomenon of interest in a qualitative systematic review).

2. The presence and description of explicit criteria for inclusion of subjects into the study.

3. The match among the clinical question, study design, and data-collection and analysis methods.

4. Evidence of any bias in the study, including selection bias (a biased distribution to groups), performance bias (different care or instructions provided that is not a part of study protocol), detection bias (uncovering group allocation), or attrition bias (loss to follow-up).

The major purpose of a critical appraisal is to select only those studies that are of the highest quality so that any recommendations made as a result of the systematic review are based on high-quality evidence. Studies retrieved for appraisal but then excluded should be reported along with the reason for exclusion. Reasons for exclusion should be related to methodology, rather than not meeting inclusion criteria.

Step 4: Construct a Table of Evidence

A Table of Evidence is a chart that displays the characteristics of all the studies included in the systematic review (Table 7.4). Each study listed in the Table of Evidence should be graded as to its level of evidence, as not all evidence is of equal value. Regardless of which grading system is used, there are commonalities across the various grading systems. The highest level of evidence is agreed to be the randomized controlled trial (referred to as Level I evidence). Next is evidence obtained from a controlled trial without randomization or evidence obtained from multiple time series with or without the intervention (referred to as Level II evidence). The third (Level III) level of evidence is obtained from observational studies, such as cohort or case-control study. The lowest grade of evidence (referred to as Level IV) is the opinion of respected authorities, based on clinical experience, case studies, or reports of expert committees.

Step 5: Interpret Results

When interpreting the results of a systematic review, it is important to consider the clinical relevance of the findings and whether the findings are precise enough to be used in point-of-care decision making. According to Burls (2009), it is imperative to determine whether there are any vital differences between the study participants and the target population that might change the effectiveness of an intervention. As Burls (2009) contends, "It is no use establishing that patients had less pain but neglecting to observe that they could be dying more often simply because this outcome was not measured" (p. 7).

The results of a systematic review of quantitative data are often reported in terms of their effect size; that is, a common metric that standardizes results across all findings so that they can be compared. An effect size is a measure of both the strength and relationship of the variables (Lipsey & Wilson, 2001). An effect size can be any statistical test. Odds ratio (OR) is the most commonly used statistical test for determining effect size with dichotomous variables (i.e., those with only two categories: yes/no, male/female). There are several statistical tests that can

TABLE 7.4 Table of Evidence

Question: What is the impact of the Synergy Model on the nurse, patient, and system outcomes?

Source	Study Purpose	Method	Design	Variables	Results	Comment
Kaplow, R. (2004). Applying the Synergy Model to nursing education. *Critical Care Nurse*, 22(Suppl. 3), 20–26.	The study linked the Synergy Model to the roles of a nurse educator. It used a case example to show how a nurse educator was able to use concepts from this model to educate a nurse in the critical care area.	Qualitative	Case study Level IV	**Nurse Competencies** Clinical judgment Advocacy Caring practices Facilitation of learning Collaboration System thinking Response to diversity Clinical inquiry **Patient Characteristics** Stability Complexity Predictability Resiliency Vulnerability Participation in decision making Resource availability	The educator used patient characteristics and nursing competencies from the Synergy Model as strategies for intervention in the mentoring/education of the nurse. This was done to enhance patient outcomes.	Patient characteristics relate to clinical condition. The educator had more (15 years) experience compared to the nurse she was mentoring. Benner's theory Novice to Expert would have provided additional support for the insight the educator had in the clinical situation. Patient outcome was used as an evaluation of this process; however, it was not clearly stated.

Source: Scarpa and Holly (2010).

be used to determine an effect size with continuous variables (i.e., those with a range of values: test scores, length of stay), including correlation coefficients and mean differences (Holly et al., 2012; Lipsey & Wilson, 2001; Littell et al., 2008). Cohen (1988) developed an often-used guide to determine whether the effect size was large, medium, or small (Table 7.5). Both the Cochran Collaboration and the Joanna Briggs Institute have available software to combine findings of individual studies and produce an effect size. The results are displayed in a forest plot, a graphic display of the results of a meta-analysis (see, e.g., Holly & Slyer, 2013).

In qualitative studies, the process of meta-synthesis is used. This involves assembling findings, categorizing the findings into groups based on similarities in meaning, and aggregating these to generate a set of synthesized statements. Figure 7.2 presents this process showing how findings are collapsed into categories after which a synthesized statement is generated.

Step 6: Report the Findings

Systematic reviews should be written according to the PRISMA guidelines (Preferred Reporting Items for Systematic Reviews and Meta-Analyses; www.prisma-statement.org). The PRISMA statement consists of a 27-item checklist and a four-phase flow diagram, and is an expansion of the now outdated QUOROM Statement. The PRISMA checklist and flow diagram are available online in both English and Spanish. Its intent is to improve the reporting of different types of health research, and in turn to improve the quality of research used in decision making in health care. The broad outline of the PRISMA statement is:

- Title, which includes the words "systematic review"
- Abstract
- Introduction with review rationale and objectives

TABLE 7.5   Cohen's Effect Sizes

Statistical Index	Large Effect	Medium Effect	Small Effect
Odds ratio used with categorical data	4.3	2.5	1.5
Standard mean difference used with continuous data	0.8	0.5	0.2

Adapted from Cohen (1988).

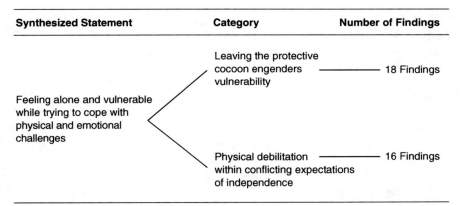

Synthesized Statement	Category	Number of Findings

FIGURE 7. 2   Findings Are Collapsed Into Categories and Categories Are Combined Into a Synthesis Statement

Source: Holly, Salmond, and Saimbert (2012).

- Method section with protocol description (eligibility criteria; appraisal method; search method; data elements to be collected, including summary methods and bias assessment)
- Results, including study selection, study characteristics, risk of bias results, results of individual studies, and synthesis of results
- Discussion, which includes a summary of results, limitations, and conclusions

CONCLUSION

Systematic reviews have been integral to the evidence-informed practice movement as a means to keep up with the ever-increasing amount of literature on a given topic (Fineout-Overholt, O'Mathuna, & Kent, 2008). However, decision makers are increasingly faced with an abundance of such reviews. Recently, the average number of systematic reviews published each day was estimated at 11. This equates to 330 each month or 3,960 per year (Bastian, Glasziou, & Chalmers, 2010; Li et al., 2012). Umbrella reviews (or overviews) of reviews are a logical and appropriate next step, allowing linkages to be formed from the findings of separate reviews. An umbrella review does not duplicate searches, assessment of eligibility, assessment of risk of bias or meta-analyses from the included reviews, but rather provides an overall picture for a particular phenomenon. This is a more useful and inclusive method of informing guidelines and clinical practice (Ionnaides, 2009).

REFLECTIVE EXERCISES

Read the following systematic review. Determine how the critical-appraisal process was conducted. Write a letter to the editor regarding the adequacy of the appraisal process.

Reisenberg, L.A., Leisch, J., & Cunningham, J. (2010). Nursing handoffs: A systematic review. *American Journal of Nursing, 110*(4), 24–34.

REFERENCES

Bastian, H., Glasziou, P., & Chalmers, I. (2010). Seventy-five trials and eleven systematic reviews a day: How will we ever keep up? *PLoS Medicine, 7*(9), e1000326.

Burls, A. (2009). *What is critical appraisal?* London, England: Hayward Medical Communications.

Chalmers, I. (2006). *The scandalous failure of scientists to cumulate scientifically* [Abstract]. Abstract to paper presented at Ninth World Congress on Health Information and Libraries, Salvador, Brazil. Retrieved from www.icml9.org/program/activity.php?lang=en&id=36

Cohen, J. (1988). *Statistical power analysis for the behavioral sciences.* New York, NY: Academic Press.

Doi, S. A., & Thalib, L. (2008). A quality-effects model for meta-analysis. *Epidemiology, 19*(1), 94–100.

Fineout-Overholt, E., O'Mathuna, D. P., & Kent, B. (2008). How systematic reviews can foster evidence-based clinical decisions. *World Views Evidence Based Nursing, 5*, 45–48.

Higgins, J. P. T., Thompson, S. G., Deeks, J. J., & Altman, D. G. (2003). Measuring inconsistency in meta-analyses. *British Medical Journal, 327*, 557–560.

Holly, C., Salmond, S., & Saimbert, M. (2012). *Comprehensive systematic review for advanced nursing practice* (p. 14). New York, NY: Springer Publishing Company.

Holly, C., & Slyer, J. (2013). Interpreting and using meta-analysis in clinical practice. *Orthopedic Nursing, 32*(2), 106–110.

Ionnaides, J. (2009). Integration of evidence from multiple meta-analyses: A primer on umbrella reviews, treatment networks and multiple treatments meta-analyses. *Canadian Medical Association Journal, 181*(8), 488–493.

Kitchenham, B. (2004). *Procedures for systematic review: Joint technical report.* Retrieved from http://csnotes.upm.edu.my/kelasmaya/pgkm20910.nsf/0/715071a8011d4c2f482577a700386d3a/$FILE/10.1.1.122.3308%5B1%5D.pdf

Li, L., Tian, J., Tian, H., Sun, R., Liu, Y., & Yang, K. (2012). Quality and transparency of overviews of systematic reviews. *Journal of Evidence-Based Medicine, 5*, 166–173.

Liberati, A., Tetzlaff, J., Altman, D. G., Mulrow, C., Gotzsche, P. C., Ioannidis, J. P., & Moher, D. (2009). Preferred reporting items for systematic reviews and meta-analyses: The PRISMA statement. *PLoS Medicine, 6*(7), e1000097. doi:10.1371/journal.pmed.1000097

Lipsey, M., & Wilson, D. (2001). *Practical meta-analysis.* Thousand Oaks, CA: Sage.

Littell, J., Corcoran, J., & Pillai, V. (2008). *Systematic reviews and meta-analysis.* New York, NY: Oxford University Press.

MetaXL. (2012). Retrieved from www.epigear.com/index_files/metaxl.html

SUGGESTED READING

Cruciani, M., & Mengoli, C. (2009). An overview of meta-analyses of diagnostic tests in infectious diseases. *Infectious Disease Clinics of North America, 23*(2), 225–267.

Hanes, K., Lockwood, C., & Pearson, A. (2010). A comparative analysis of three appraisal instruments to assess validity in qualitative research. *Qualitative Health Research, 20*(12), 1736–1743.

Holly, C., Cantwell, E. R., & Kamienski, M. (2013). Evidence-based practices for the identification, screening, and prevention of acute delirium in the hospitalized elderly: An overview of systematic reviews. *Current Translational Geriatrics and Experimental Gerontology Reports, 2*(1), 7–15.

Holly, C., & Slyer, J. (2013). Interpreting and using meta-analysis in clinical practice. *Orthopedic Nursing, 32*(2), 106–110.

Pearson, A., Wiechula, R., Court, A., & Lockwood, C. (2005). The JBI model of evidence-based healthcare. *International Journal of Evidence-Based Healthcare, 3*, 207–215.

A Systematic Review of the Effectiveness of Three Methods of Fentanyl Administration Following Discharge From Acute Care

MARYANNE M. GIULIANTE
ANGELITO S. ANTONIO
KEESHA A. DUNCAN

Background: There are nearly 1.5 million new cases of cancer diagnosed annually, with estimates of up to 80% of these patients diagnosed with advanced cancer and inadequately controlled moderate to severe pain (American Cancer Society, 2011). Achieving effective pain control in this population can be demanding and present inherent challenges related to mode of administration. Determining timely and effective treatment of pain is the cornerstone in management of cancer pain with the goal focused on maintaining quality of life. Fluctuations in the pain, variability of accurate reporting, psychosocial underpinnings, addictive potential, and common side effects make this type of pain management challenging. Although opioids are the standard for cancer pain management, fentanyl, available for administration via several modalities, including intravenously, transdermally, buccally, nasally, and submucosally, has a clinical potency ratio 50 to 100 times that of morphine and has grown in popularity for cancer pain management.

Aims: The primary aim of this systematic review was to examine the evidence on the effectiveness of fentanyl modalities for the adult cancer patient. Modes of administration reviewed were: transdermal, buccal, intranasal, and oral transmucosal. A secondary aim of the review was to describe cost utility and cost-effectiveness among various modes of fentanyl administration.

Method: An exhaustive literature review was conducted to capture all applicable data. The search strategy aimed to find both published and unpublished studies. A four-step search strategy was used in this review. First, a limited search of MEDLINE and CINAHL was undertaken using the keywords "fentanyl," "adult cancer patient," and "chronic pain management." This was followed by an analysis of the text words contained in the title and abstract of all identified papers. A second search using the expanded list was then undertaken across all included databases. Third, the reference lists of all articles were searched for additional studies. Studies published in the English language and available in full text were considered for inclusion in this review. Finally, five journals specific to the topic were hand searched. These included *AANA Journal, Pain and Analgesia Journal, Journal of Pharmacology, Nurse Economics,* and *Cancer Nursing.*

Two reviewers independently assessed all studies identified from the search strategy against the inclusion criteria. Any disagreements that arose between the reviewers were resolved through discussion or with a third reviewer until consensus was reached. In the second step, all studies that were deemed relevant were retrieved for a full text review. These articles were also reviewed by two independent reviewers to establish whether the study met the inclusion criteria. Those studies that did not meet the inclusion criteria were excluded from the systematic review and recorded in a list of exclusion. In the third step, studies that met the inclusion criteria were further assessed for methodological quality using standardized critical-appraisal instruments.

Results: We identified 711 potential studies. Of these, 16 studies were retrieved for appraisal and 11 are included in this review: 9 randomized controlled trials on the effectiveness of fentanyl and 2 on the economics of fentanyl use (one cost-utility study and one cost-effectiveness study). Due to heterogeneity, a meta-analysis was not possible, and studies were presented as a narrative.

Findings: The findings of this review suggest that fentanyl provides adequate pain relief alone, and may be more effective than other methods studied, such as tramadol, methadone, Dilaudid, or morphine, in relieving pain in the adult cancer patient. Fentanyl in spray form had a more rapid onset than other drugs used for breakthrough pain (Level I). Fentanyl was found to be cost-effective and increased quality of life (Level II).

Conclusion: Given the availability of various modalities of administration, fentanyl use is logistically feasible when practitioners are challenged by the inability to use an oral route for pain relief.

Integrative Review

OBJECTIVES

At the end of this chapter, you will be able to:
- Differentiate among a review of the literature, an integrative review, and a systematic review
- Determine which of the reviews will best answer your question
- Describe the steps to conduct an integrative review of the literature

KEY CONCEPTS

- An integrative review of the literature is a summary of available evidence.
- Rigorous integrative reviews can contribute to theory development.
- Integrative reviews are useful for keeping current with the ever-expanding volume of literature.
- Integrative reviews summarize what is known at a particular point in time.

An integrative review is not a research method; nor can an integrative review of the literature be used as a synonym for a literature review, systematic review, or a meta-analysis. See Table 8.1 for a comparison of these review methods. An integrative literature review summarizes the main points of past research to draw general conclusions from a literary source on a certain topic using literature that includes studies that address related or identical hypotheses (unipapers.org/guide/integrative-literature-review). Essentially, it is a critical summary of literature on a particular topic. As such, an integrative review appraises and combines available evidence, including theory. The integrative review method can incorporate diverse methodologies to capture the circumstances, processes, and individual elements of the topic under study (Whittemore & Knafl, 2005). It takes a traditional review of the literature one step further by providing a more substantial contribution

125

TABLE 8.1 Types of Review

	Literature Review	Integrative Review	Systematic Review
Focus	Broad	Defined	Precise
Search strategy	Limited to 5 years. May include a search of only one database or search engine	Based on keywords. Searches for pivotal papers in 2–6 databases or search engines	Exhaustive, including hand searching and search for unpublished (grey) literature; uses an explicit strategy
Appraisal	Appraisal is done to establish support for research question	Appraisal may be rigorous, but may be done by only one reviewer	Rigorous appraisal by two independent reviewers; uses valid and reliable tools for appraisal based on the study research design
Outcome	Background	Recommendations	Best practice

to knowledge using a transparent process, and may also involve a critical appraisal of the literature used in the review. New perspectives and frameworks can be generated through an integrative review, and research questions can be developed. An integrative review of the literature has a broader focus than a traditional review of the literature, but not the focused clinical question associated with a systematic review. There are many benefits to an integrative review, including:

- Definition of concepts
- Review and comparison of theories
- Analysis of methodological issues on a particular topic
- Accentuation of unresolved issues or gaps in knowledge
- Identification of trends
- Evaluation of current practices

Conducting an integrative literature review involves the same rigor used when conducting primary research. At first, there are four questions to ask when considering an integrative review of the literature (Russell, 2011):

- What is known?
- What is the quality of what is known?
- What should be known?
- What is the next step for research or practice?

STEPS IN AN INTEGRATIVE REVIEW

Step 1: Selecting the Question or Hypothesis for Review

The task of developing guiding questions to focus the review is of immense importance. These questions provide direction for all other phases of the review. As discussed in Chapter 2, the questions should flow from the aim or purpose of the review. See Box 8.1 for an example. Key concepts such as the population for study, any interventions of interest, comparison groups, and outcomes should be evident in the guiding questions. Well-stated guiding questions will help to resolve any ambiguity in the review and facilitate in delineating the scope of the review (Broome, 2000).

The scope, or range, of the review is very important. If a number of studies have been conducted on the question of interest, the reviewer needs to narrow the question. On the other hand, if the topic has little research available, the question may need to be expanded. Russell (2005) provides this example:

> If the reviewer's initial research question is "What interventions are most effective in increasing treatment compliance in liver transplant recipients?" but no intervention studies have been conducted with this population, then the reviewer may need

---

Box 8.1

EXAMPLE OF GUIDING QUESTIONS FOR AN INTEGRATIVE REVIEW

The objective of this integrative review was to examine the evidence on factors that influence, and strategies that support, the academic success of culturally diverse students. Specifically, the questions that guided the review were:

1. What are the facilitators and barriers to successful completion of a nursing program for culturally diverse students?
2. What are the strategies that support success in NCLEX-RN® (National Council Licensure Examination for Registered Nurses) examination for culturally diverse students?
3. What are the characteristics of successful retention programs for culturally diverse students?

Adapted from Cantwell and Holly (2012).

to broaden the research question to, "What interventions are the most effective in increasing treatment compliance in all transplant recipients?" (p. 2)

Step 2: Locating the Right Studies for Inclusion in the Review

The search for the right studies to include in the integrative review is part of the data-collection phase. Using the keywords and phrases garnered from the guiding questions, a search strategy is developed. The search should be broad and encompass a minimum of two databases, although a search of three to six databases is preferred. This search of databases is different from a systematic review, in which as many databases as necessary are searched so that the examination is exhaustive. The strategy developed should include an electronic database search, a hand search in journals relevant to the guiding questions, and a search of the reference list of studies selected to be in the review. A search for grey or unpublished literature can be considered. Also, authors who have previously published on the topic for review can be contacted to determine whether any other sources are available. At the end of the search, the reviewer should have in hand all of the evidence that could potentially be used in the review.

Some of the common databases that can be searched for an integrative review on a nursing topic include:

1. Academic Search Premier, which contains indexing and abstracts for more than 8,500 journals, with full text for more than 4,600 of those titles related to health, medicine, and biology, among others. It also contains author contact information that can be useful in identifying other relevant studies for inclusion in the review.

2. MEDLINE/PubMed (Medical Literature Analysis and Retrieval System Online), a database of life sciences and biomedical information compiled by the National Library of Medicine. It includes information for articles from academic journals covering medicine, nursing, pharmacy, dentistry, veterinary medicine, and health care.

3. CINAHL, a database of nursing and allied health literature with indexing for more than 3,000 journals and more than 2.6 million records dating back to 1981. In addition, this database offers access to health care books, nursing dissertations, selected conference proceedings, standards of practice, educational software, audiovisuals, and book chapters.

4. Web of Science, an online academic citation index provided by Thomson Reuters. It allows access to multiple databases for cross-disciplinary research and in-depth exploration of specialized subfields within an academic or scientific discipline. As a citation index, any cited paper will lead to any other literature (book, academic journal, proceedings, etc.) that currently, or in the past, cites this work.

5. Mednar, a free, publicly available search engine that does deep web searches. It includes a search of the Cochrane Library, Google Scholar, MEDLINE/PubMed, and all National Institutes of Health (NIH) websites.

The search should involve seeking primary, secondary, and tertiary literature. Primary literature is an original study, or primary research. For example, Hartog et al. (2010) studied the neurological outcomes of patients admitted to an intensive care unit with temperatures below 35°C. Secondary literature summarizes and synthesizes primary literature. Secondary literature includes meta-analysis, meta-syntheses, and systematic review. Textbooks are also considered secondary literature. Completed secondary literature reports can be found in the Cochrane (www.cochrane.org) or the Joanna Briggs Library (www.joannabrigg.edu.au). Tertiary literature is a summary or an abstract of primary or secondary literature. Online databases such as WebMD (www.webmd.com) or Dynamed (dynamed.ebscohost.com) are tertiary literature sites (Holly, Salmond, & Saimbert, 2012).

Step 3: Representing the Findings of the Studies

To assist in having a review that contains only the best available evidence, each of the selected studies needs to be critically appraised. Holly et al. (2012) have noted that "The critical appraisal provides a balanced assessment of the benefits and strengths of the research against its flaws and weaknesses" (p. 148). The focus in a critical appraisal is on the validity, reliability, and rigor of the study. Studies not meeting the appraisal criteria are excluded. *Validity* refers to the legitimacy of the findings; in other words, how authentic, truthful, and accurate they are. *Reliability* refers to the consistency of the findings, and *rigor* refers to the exactness with which the research study was designed. To determine how valid, reliable, and rigorous a study is, papers need to be read several times when doing a critical appraisal. Greenhalgh (2006) reminds us that the goal of critical appraisal is not finding methodologically flawless papers, for in reality there are flaws in 99% of all research studies. Rather, the aim is to identify papers that are "good enough." In other words, those papers that meet the indicators believed to show quality can be considered good enough.

Critical appraisal for an integrative review can be completed by one investigator. In comparison, a critical appraisal for a systematic review must be completed by two reviewers working independently. A review of the literature generally does not undergo a critical appraisal.

A detailed log of the papers determined not to be good enough should be kept and the reason for exclusion noted.

An appraisal focuses on adequacy of reporting of data-collection methods, appropriate data analysis, and whether key findings were reported appropriately. Questions to ask when determining whether a study is appropriate for an integrative review include:

- Is the study question relevant to my guiding questions and target population?
- Does the study add anything new or support current thinking or theory on the topic?
- Was the study design appropriate for the research question?
- Did the study methods address the most important potential sources of bias? These can include selection bias (a differential selection of subjects for comparison groups), attrition (loss of subjects to follow-up), or instrumentation (changes in calibration of a measurement tool or changes in the observers or scorers that can produce changes in the outcome measured).
- Was the appropriate analytic method chosen and was it performed correctly?
- Are the conclusions based on the data?

Alternately, a critical appraisal tool, such as those developed by the Critical Skills Appraisal Programme (CASP), can be used. These appraisal tools are based on the research study design and can be accessed for free (www.sph.nhs.uk/what-we-do/public-health-workforce/resources/critical-appraisals-skills-programme).

When the critical appraisal has been completed, a table can be created that contains information about each of the studies in the review. Called a table of inclusion, it should contain information about:

- The author, title, and source of the paper
- Purpose of the study
- Study design

- Sample size and major characteristics
- How the data were collected and analyzed
- Major findings
- Comments

Step 4: Analyzing the Findings

The findings of studies that have been appraised and are to be used in the study next need to be extracted. To guarantee relevancy and accuracy when extracting data from a selected study, a tool should be used. Extracted data should include definition of the subjects, methodology, size of the sample, variables, method of analysis, and results. Categories and data-display matrices are then developed to display all of the coded data from each study by its category. Next, these are iteratively compared. As data are conceptualized at higher and higher levels of abstraction, each primary source is re-read and reviewed to verify that the new conceptualization was congruent with primary sources. For a detailed description of this process, see Whittemore and Knafl (2005).

Step 5: Summarizing Results

Drawing conclusions and summarizing results is the final step in an integrative review, and is generally done as a narrative. Similarities and differences in the findings are identified with a description of generalizations representative of the defined categories and the integrative review in its entirety, as possible (Whittemore & Knafl, 2005). Findings can be presented as a research agenda, a conceptual model, or a taxonomy (see Table 8.2).

TABLE 8.2   Outcomes of an Integrative Review

A research agenda that flows logically from the critical analysis of the literature. The research agenda should pose provocative questions (or propositions) that give direction for future research.

A taxonomy developed as a means to classify previous research and can contribute to the research agenda.

Conceptual framework or new ways of thinking about the topic can be developed.

Adapted from Torraco (2005).

REPORTING THE INTEGRATIVE REVIEW

There is no one standard template for reporting integrative research reviews. A suggested format is to follow the general outline used for primary research, which includes introduction, methods, results, and discussion sections. This should be a fully synthesized report showing the themes derived across studies. The introduction should include the list of guiding questions developed for the review and definitions of the conceptual and operational variables that were a part of the review. The method section should be transparent in its description of the search strategy used to locate the papers included in the review. An example of the search strategy should be included in a table or in an appendix. The approach to analyzing the data and generating themes or categories should be described. The results section should summarize and synthesize the themes that were uncovered in the review. Finally, in the discussion section, inferences should be drawn and discussed in relation to the guiding questions.

CONCLUSION

The integrative literature review has many benefits to a scholarly inquiry, including identifying gaps in current research, evaluating the strength of available research, and providing a strong foundation for primary research studies. Although it is not a research method, an integrative review can provide important information for the conduct of primary or translational studies.

REFLECTIVE EXERCISES

1. When discharged patients transition from the acute care settings back to their community, follow-up by home health care nurses may be necessary to prevent readmission. Write the guiding question for an integrative review of heart failure patients who are transitioning back to the community and who are being followed by a home health care nurse. What would the nurse need to know and what follow-up strategies would she use? Then devise a search strategy to find papers relevant to this topic.

2. Read the following integrative review. What are the findings of the review? Using these findings, write research questions that can be used to conduct a primary study on this topic.

Alekseyev, S., Byrne, M., Carpenter, A., Franker, C., Kidd, C., & Hulton, L. (2012). Prolonging the life of a patient's IV: An integrative review of intravenous securement devices. *Medsurg Nursing, 21*(5), 285–292.

REFERENCES

Broome, M. E. (2000). Integrative literature reviews for the development of concepts. In B. Rogers & K. Knafl (Eds.), *Concept development in nursing* (pp. 231–250). Philadelphia, PA: Saunders.

Cantwell, E. R., & Holly, C. (2012). *An integrative review on the best strategies to assist culturally diverse nursing students toward successful program completion.* Unpublished manuscript.

Greenhalgh, T. (2006). *How to read a paper.* Chichester, England: Wiley.

Hartog, A., dePont, A., Robillard, L., Binnekade, J., Schultz, M., & Horn, J. (2010). Spontaneous hypothermia on intensive care unit admission is a predictor of unfavorable neurological outcome in patients after resuscitation: An observational cohort study. *Critical Care, 14,* R121.

Holly, C., Salmond, S., & Saimbert, M. (2012). *Comprehensive systematic review for advanced nursing practice.* New York, NY: Springer Publishing Company.

Russell, C. L. (2005). *An overview of the integrative research review. Progress in transplantation.* Retrieved from http://www.nitiphong.com/paper_pdf/phd/ An%20overview%20of%20the%20integrative%20research%20review.pdf

Torraco, R. J. (2005). Writing integrative literature reviews: Guidelines and examples. *Human Resource Development Review, 4,* 356. Retrieved from http://hrd.sagepub.com/content/4/3/356

Whittemore, R., & Knafl, K. (2005). The integrative review: Updated methodology. *Journal of Advanced Nursing, 52*(5), 546–553.

SUGGESTED READING

Reid, V., & Meadows-Oliver, M. (2007). Postpartum depression in adolescent mothers: An integrative review of the literature. *Journal of Pediatric Health Care, 21*(5), 289–298. doi: 10.1016/j.pedhc.2006.05.010

Sulosaari, V., Suhonen, R., & Leino-Kilp, H. (2011). An integrative review of the literature on registered nurses' medication competence. *Journal of Clinical Nursing, 20*(3–4), 464–478.

Young, J., & Solomon, M. (2009). How to critically appraise an article. *Nature Clinical Practice Gastroenterology and Hepatology, 6*(2), 82–91.

An Integrative Review as the Foundation for Development of a Medication Safety Program for Undergraduate Nursing Students

JACKELINE BIDDLE SHULER

Background: Medication errors are substantially responsible for morbidity and mortality costing in excess of billions of dollars. Communication failure is a significant cause of these errors. Situation, Background, Assessment, and Recommendation (SBAR) is a standardized approach of communication that has been found to be effective because it creates redundancy in how information is transmitted. The literature identifies SBAR as best practice as a communication improvement tool because it has features of approaches used by high-reliability organizations such as the airline industry. The goal of standardizing medication communication is to reduce the risk of medication error and to engage prospective nurses in medication safety awareness. Baccalaureate nursing students must be prepared to improve medication safety, as on average nurses in hospitals spend about 40% of their time administering medications.

Aims: To conduct an integrative review of the literature related to medication communication, medication safety, and the use of SBAR in an acute care context; to design a medication safety program focusing on improving communication; to recommend practices for incorporating medication safety into prelicensure programs.

Method: The design used an integrative review of the literature that served to support the development of a medication safety program. An integrative review is defined as a broad method of research that includes the simultaneous review of experimental and nonexperimental research to explore a health care issue. The methodology involved a review of all relevant available qualitative, quantitative, and mixed-methods studies, including published and grey literature from the time period between 2000 and 2013. The integrative review followed a five-step, evidence-based process that included the following: *Step 1: Problem Identification,* wherein the review was guided by questions developed using the population, intervention, comparison, outcomes (PICO) approach; *Step 2: Literature Search,* wherein keywords were used to acquire evidence via an electronic search, a hand search, and the search of reference lists; *Step 3: Data Appraisal,* wherein a valid and reliable appraisal tool was used for verification of methodological quality; *Step 4: Data Extraction,* wherein the appraised evidence was applied to the project via use of a table of evidence that was used as a data-extraction tool, which included the source, study purpose, study design, discussion, and level of evidence, and themes were generated; and *Step 5: Implement and Evaluate,* wherein the lesson plan was developed as per the evidence and reviewed by an expert review panel that included nursing faculty who taught pharmacology with a background in risk management.

Results: The initial search found 350 relevant articles. After a review of the title and abstract, 77 were retrieved for appraisal and 31 were included in this review. Three themes were generated through the integrative review: (a) Improving medication safety involves attention to communication and team relationships; (b) the use of SBAR (situation–background–assessment–recommendation) increases students' confidence and willingness to report to colleagues; and (c) enhanced communication skills reduce medication errors.

Outcomes: The findings of the integrative review were used to develop a plan for a medication safety program titled "Communication is Key: Using SBAR for Medication Safety." The program was reviewed by an expert panel of DNP and PhD nursing faculty for feasibility and applicability, who provided recommendations for improvement. The review panel evaluated the plan and determined it to be feasible to implement and applicable to current nursing practice. Recommendations about the lesson's objectives, teaching content, teaching strategies, time allotment, and evaluation were incorporated into the plan. The objectives of the medication safety program are to: (a) define the attributes of effective communication, (b) identify primary factors in communication failure, (c) describe the challenges associated with administration of medication in acute care settings, (d) explain how a communication improvement strategy can enhance medication safety, and (e) demonstrate the use of SBAR.

9

Quality Improvement

OBJECTIVES

At the end of this chapter, you will be able to:
- Define quality improvement
- Differentiate between quality-improvement studies and research studies
- Select a method for a quality-improvement study
- Determine the appropriate quality-management tool to assess outcomes

KEY CONCEPTS

- Quality implies a continuous monitoring process.
- Quality improvement is a focus on the structure, process, and outcomes of health care.
- Quality improvement has its own validated methods and tools for analysis.

Quality is an abstract concept conceptualized as a balance among possibilities, norms, and values, rather than a discrete entity (Harteloh, 2003; Mitchell, 2008). According to Donabedian (1990), seven attributes of health care define its quality: (a) efficacy: the ability of care to improve health; (b) effectiveness: how well health improvements are realized; (c) efficiency: the facility to obtain the best health improvement at the lowest cost; (d) optimality: balancing costs and benefits; (e) acceptability: taking into account patient preferences; (f) legitimacy: accord with social preferences concerning all of the above; and (g) equity: fair distribution of care (p. 1115).

To achieve quality, it is necessary to have data-guided activities for improvement in health care delivery (Lynn et al., 2007) and to define and understand the issues that are hindering quality (Neuhauser, Myhre, & Alemi, 2004). These strategies include "any intervention aimed at reducing the quality gap for a group of patients representative of those encountered in routine practice" (Shojania et al., 2004, p. 13). For example, automatic triggers can be set in an electronic medical record to remind staff to check blood glucose levels at a specific time.

Quality-improvement projects are not research studies, although the scientific method may be used. Quality-improvement projects carry no risk to patients and are meant to be generalizable only within the setting in which the project was conducted. Research, on the other hand, is a systematic investigation meant to generate generalizable knowledge. Ask the following questions to determine whether the project is a research study or a quality-improvement project (Johansson, 2011; Platteborze et al., 2010; Reinhardt & Ray, 2003):

1. Quality-Improvement Project
   - Are patients involved only through the use of a medical record review?
   - Are data being reviewed to correct deficiencies or improve a process?
   - Is there a continuous monitoring process?
   - Are a set of standards, benchmarks, or guidelines used for comparison?
   - Is immediate feedback provided to stakeholders during and after the project?
2. Research Study
   - Are interventions being tested?
   - Were patients allocated to different groups for monitoring or testing?
   - Is anyone blinded to the patients involved or procedure or testing being done?
   - Was feedback deliberately delayed?
   - Was statistical testing done to prove or disprove a hypothesis?

DETERMINING QUALITY MEASURES

The focus of quality-improvement activities is on systems and processes that can be improved. According to Glanville, Schrim, and Wineman (2000), the classic five Ds of medical outcomes are a starting point. The five Ds are: death, disease, disability, discomfort, and dissatisfaction. Examples of processes and systems amenable to quality improvement using this framework include:

- Infant mortality; serious drug errors; death while under anesthesia in the operating room (death)
- Quality of life, for example, improved balance for those with multiple sclerosis (disability)

- Urinary tract infections, readmission rates for heart failure (disease)
- Pain, pressure ulcers (discomfort)
- Hospital noise levels at night; staffing mix; turnover rates; waiting times (dissatisfaction)

Donabedian (2003) described three key aspects to an understanding of quality in health care, which can be used to determine quality indicators for monitoring. These are structure, process, and outcomes. Structure is the environment in which care is provided, and includes material resources, human resources (e.g., care provider qualifications), and organizational resources. Data on structure variables are usually readily available.

Process refers to the way in which health care services are provided, including the individual decisions and performance of those rendering care. Process variables examine the appropriateness and completeness of care rendered. Often process variables are categorized as quality care (e.g., infection rates), safety (e.g., fall rates), or communication (e.g., discharge teaching).

Outcomes are the products that result from the interaction of structure and process. The outcome reflects what was done to a patient and how well it was done. Outcomes, as the endpoint of care, can be expected or unexpected; desirable or undesirable. Death, disability, satisfaction, length of stay, readmission rates, and cost are examples of outcome variables.

According to Donabedian (2003), examining structure, process, and outcomes as an integrated whole provides a comprehensive review of quality care. For example, when a structure, process, or outcome has been determined to be in need of improvement, it is weighted more heavily if it has one or more of the following characteristics (Health Resources and Services Administration, 2011):

- High volume
- High frequency
- High risk
- Long-standing
- Multiple unsuccessful attempts to resolve the issue in the past
- Strong and differing opinions on cause or resolution of the problem

METHODS FOR QUALITY IMPROVEMENT

Several models exist for use in quality improvement, as presented in Table 9.1. Among these are Plan–Do–Check–Act (PDCA), Six Sigma, Baldrige, LEAN, and ISO 9000. The two most frequently used are PDCA and Six Sigma.

TABLE 9.1   Quality-Improvement Methods

Method	Key Components	Learn More
Baldrige	The Baldrige program consists of a set of 18 performance criteria divided into 7 categories: 1. leadership 2. strategic excellence: focus on patients 3. other customers and markets 4. measurement, analysis, and knowledge management 5. workforce focus 6. process management 7. results	www.qualitynist.gov Flynn, B., & Saladin, B. (2001). Further evidence on the validity of the theoretical models underlying the Baldrige criteria. *Journal of Operations Management, 19*(6), 617–652.
ISO 9000	The ISO 9000 is a set of eight standards developed to align organizational goals, communication, and continuous improvement. The standards focus on: 1. customers 2. leadership 3. involvement of people 4. process 5. systems 6. continual improvement 7. factual approach to decision making 8. supplier relationships	www.vmiso.org Sweeney, J., & Heaton, C. (2000). Interpretations and variations of ISO 9000 in acute health care. *International Journal of Quality Health Care, 12*(3), 203–209.
Six Sigma	Six Sigma is a process designed to eliminate variation and reduce the likelihood of error and streamlining processes.	www isixsigma.org Lanham, B., & Maxson-Cooper, P. (2003). Is Six Sigma the answer for nursing to reduce medical errors and enhance patient safety? *Nursing Economics, 21*(1), 39–41.

(continued)

TABLE 9.1   Quality-Improvement Methods (*continued*)

Method	Key Components	Learn More
LEAN	The basis of LEAN management is determining the value of a given process by breaking it down and identifying the value-added steps and the non–value-added steps. A central element is "stop the line," which allows any employee to stop a process when a defect is identified or suspected.	www.ihi.org IHI/Results/WhitePapers/GoingLeaninHealthCare.htm Furman, C., & Caplan, R. (2007). Applying the Toyota production system: Using a patient safety alert system to reduce error. *Joint Commission Journal on Quality and Patient Safety,* *33*(7), 376–386.
PDCA	Plan–Do–Check–Act (PDCA) is a four-step cyclical process involving establishing objectives and outcome, developing an implementation strategy, implementing the plan, and evaluating the results.	www.ihi.org van Tiel, F. H., Elenbaas, T. W., Voskuilen, B. M., Herczeg, J., Verheggen, F. W., Mochtar, B., & Stobberingh, E. E. (2006). Plan-do-study-act cycles as an instrument for improvement of compliance with infection control measures in care of patients after cardiothoracic surgery. *Journal of Hospital Infections, 62,* 64–70.

PDCA is a four-step iterative process. The first step is to identify the problem and formulate an approach to resolving it (*Plan*) by establishing objectives and expected outcomes; for example, a reduction in catheter-associated urinary tract infections or reduction in readmission rates to a detoxification facility. Second, the plan is implemented (*Do*), and data are collected. The Do phase often incorporates such processes as LEAN and Six Sigma. LEAN focuses on understanding and improving processes, whereas Six Sigma seeks to uncover and reduce variation (Langley, Nolan, Nolan, Norman, & Procost, 2009). The Do phase is the most extensive and time-consuming as protocols and tools are being developed or refined and often an educational component is necessary to instruct staff on any new processes or protocols. Third, collected data are analyzed and compared with the goals and expectations devised during the Plan phase (*Check*). Quality-improvement tools, such as flowcharts, Pareto charts, or control charts, are used to display and interpret data. Finally, the plan is refined and further improvements are made as necessary or strategies are put into place to sustain and monitor positive outcomes (*Act*). Both failures and successes are analyzed in this phase. Corrective action plans can be devised for differences in the project goals and results or a root cause analysis can be conducted for major differences or lack of goal attainment.

Six Sigma is a method used to investigate operational performance improvement. It is a five-step process of defining, measuring, analyzing, improving, and controlling (DMAIC; Corn, 2009). For example, if the staff in a psychiatric rehabilitation facility believes it has a high rate of transfer to local emergency departments for minor ailments among its residents, a team will first delineate the problem (*Define*). This can be done by reviewing the transfer records of all patients taken to the emergency department for a specified period of time. This review will provide information on the scope of the problem, such as common reasons for transfer and cost. Second, the team will determine measures to define its success in reducing rates of transfer. Goals should be written to keep the project on track (*Measure*). For example, reduce transfers to the emergency department by two per month over the next 6 months. Next, the team will need to analyze each of the transfers to determine the reason for each transfer and if it were an actual emergency, as well as other information that will inform development of a plan for improvement, for example, dates and times of transfer, staffing mix at times of transfer (*Analyze*). Use of the quality-management tools, such as the Pareto chart, can better inform this analysis (see the section "Pareto Chart"). A plan to address the process is then developed (*Improve*); for example, staff education on minor versus major emergencies, review of medical coverage or need for additional coverage (medical as well as psychiatric coverage) at certain times. Finally, the plan will need constant monitoring over time with feedback provided to staff and administrators so that progress can be monitored (*Control*). Here, the quality-management tool, the control chart, can be used to monitor process control (see the section "Control Chart"). This model can be used in conjunction with a root cause analysis.

Two other frequently used strategies for quality improvement are the root cause analysis (RCA) and failure mode effect analysis. An RCA is a formal team investigation aimed at identifying and understanding why an event occurred. The team should include at a minimum: stakeholders with decisional authority, a clinician with knowledge of the processes and procedures, and a quality-improvement expert (American Society for Quality [ASQ], 2013). An RCA is undertaken with the understanding that system issues, rather than personnel, are likely the source of an incident. According to Hughes (2008), an RCA is a labor-intensive assessment that begins after an event occurs (e.g., a death while under anesthesia in the operating room, or the suicide of a patient on a psychiatric unit). The process involves tracing and outlining the sequence of events leading to the event and putting preventive strategies into place. Meetings of the team should focus on defining and understanding the problem, brainstorming its possible causes, analyzing causes and effects, and devising a solution to the problem (ASQ, 2013). RCA uses qualitative methods of inquiry, including interviewing those involved in the event. Interview questions are focused on enabling factors (e.g., lack of education), latent conditions (e.g., not checking the patient's identification band), and situational factors (e.g., two patients in the hospital with the same last name) that contributed to or enabled the adverse event. It is important to continually ask "Why did this happen?" until the root cause or causes are determined. It is important to also consider events that occurred immediately prior to the event to determine whether any other factors may have contributed (The Joint Commission [TJC], 2003). The final step of an RCA is developing recommendations into a plan of corrective action.

A second commonly used strategy is a *failure modes and effects analysis* (FMEA). This is an evaluation strategy to identify and eliminate failures before they actually occur. In other words, identifying the parts of a process that need to be strengthened or improved before an adverse event occurs. The goal of FMEA is to prevent errors by attempting to identify the ways a process could fail, estimate the probability and consequences of each failure, and then take action to prevent the potential failures from occurring (Hughes, 2008). Brainstorming and speculation are important activities in this process. The ASQ (2013) suggests that an FMEA be considered for any of the following:

- When a new service is being designed or implemented
- When an existing process is used in a new way
- When analyzing failures of an existing process
- Periodically to monitor change over time

The focus of the analysis is on the steps in the process, failure modes (What could go wrong?), failure causes (Why would the failure happen?), and failure effects (What would be the consequences of each failure?; Institute for Healthcare Improvement [IHI], 2011). The IHI (2004) has an interactive tool to assist in the conduct of an FMEA. Use of this tool allows a risk score to be generated that takes into account the likelihood that the process will actually fail, the potential to detect the failure, and the severity of a failure.

TOOLS FOR QUALITY IMPROVEMENT

There are several tools that can be used for displaying and monitoring the results of quality-improvement initiatives. The most commonly used are:

- Flowchart
- Fishbone
- Run chart
- Pareto chart
- Control chart

The technique of brainstorming, however, is foundational to all of these improvement tools. Brainstorming is a group method of discussing a problem or clinical issue and a list of broad-ranging ideas on the topic. It is meant to be a creative and open process with little structure so that a complete list of potential causes can be generated. All suggestions are put into a list. To be successful, a brainstorming session should have a leader who presents and clarifies the issue for discussion and one (or more) recorder who puts all ideas onto a flip chart or white board. Also important to a brainstorming session is an understanding that this is not a debate on how best to address a problem; rather, it is an open discussion of the issue. See Box 9.1 for other resources to manage quality data.

Box 9.1

RESOURCES FOR MANAGING QUALITY DATA

1. Institute for Healthcare Improvement. (2011). *Simple data collection planning.* www.ihi.org/knowledge/Pages/Tools/ SimpleDataCollectionPlanning.aspx
2. Agency for Healthcare Research and Quality. (2010). *Introduction to measures of quality.* www.ahrq.gov/professionals/ quality-patient-safety/quality-resources/perfmeasguide/ perfmeaspt2.html
3. Agency for Healthcare Research and Quality. (2011). *National Quality Measures Clearinghouse.* www.qualitymeasures .ahrq.gov/search/advanced-search.aspx
4. Institute for Healthcare Improvement. (2011). *Sampling tool for quality management.* www.ihi.org/knowledge/ Pages/Tools/Sampling.aspx

---

(continued)

(continued)

5. Institute for Healthcare Improvement. (2011). *Improvement tracker.* app.ihi.org/Workspace/tracker
6. Institute for Healthcare Improvement. (2011). *Plan-do-study-act worksheet.* www.ihi.org/knowledge/Pages/Tools/Plan DoStudyActWorksheet.aspx
7. American Society for Quality. (2004). *When to use a check sheet for observations.* asq.org/learn-about-quality/data-collection-analysis-tools/overview/check-sheet.html
8. Health Resources and Services Administration. (2011). *Quality management toolkit.* www.hrsa.gov/quality/tool-box/index.html

Flowchart

A flowchart is a schematic representation of a process that allows visualization of the steps in a process. Each step is represented by a different symbol and contains a short description of the process step. Once the steps in a process are identified, the flowchart can be used to identify unnecessary or duplicative steps, missing steps, and integration among the steps. The most common types of boxes in a flowchart are an oval, which indicates the starting and ending points of a process; a rectangle, which denotes an activity or a step in the process; and a diamond, which is a decision point. The flowchart symbols are linked together with arrows showing the process-flow direction. Flowcharts can be constructed in Microsoft Excel, Word, or PowerPoint. Common alternate names include: process flowchart, process map, process chart, process model, process flow diagram, or just flow diagram. Flowcharts are useful in detailing the steps of a procedure or a process; for example, how pressure ulcers are assessed (see Figure 9.1).

Fishbone

A fishbone diagram is a graphic display of the possible causes or effects of a quality issue. It can be used to summarize a brainstorming session. Often, it is constructed following the development of a flowchart when all processes are understood. It can also be used following an adverse event to determine the cause of the event or to determine any potential problems in a process (root cause analysis). Fishbones are categorized into manpower (people), material, machinery (equipment), measurement, and methods. Environment may also be added if appropriate.

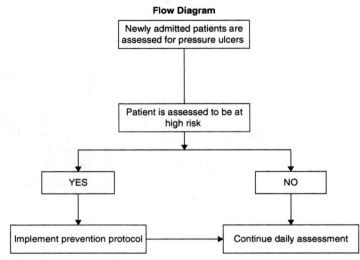

FIGURE 9.1   Sample Flowchart

Each of these categories forms a bone in the fish. Fishbone diagrams are also referred to as cause-and-effect diagrams or Ishikawa diagrams (see Figure 9.2). Other areas in need of brainstorming can be added, such as environment or generic headings.

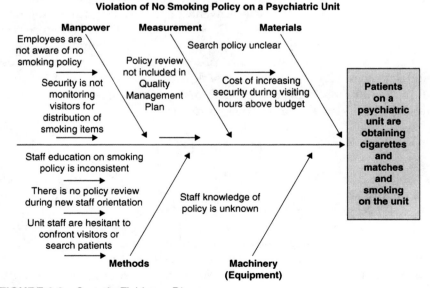

FIGURE 9.2   Sample Fishbone Diagram

Run Chart

Run charts, or line graphs, display results and variation over time and in time sequence. In a run chart, events, shown on the y (vertical) axis, are graphed against a time period, shown on the x (horizontal) axis. For example, a run chart can plot the time of a written discharge order to the actual time the patient leaves the hospital room. The results might show that although the order is written in the morning, patients do not leave until late afternoon. Investigating this phenomenon could identify areas for potential improvement in the discharge process. As an example, Figure 9.3 presents a run chart used to plot the number of falls per month in order to detect whether the number is increasing, decreasing, or remaining the same over time.

Pareto Chart

The Pareto chart is a clustered bar chart with values arranged in order of frequency of occurrence and percentage of the total represented by each of the frequencies. A Pareto chart identifies the most significant factors in a quality issue by using the 80/20 question: What 20% is causing 80% of a problem? For example, although there may be many patient complaints about the food served in a hospital, a Pareto chart helps identify the most common complaints and where efforts to reduce complaint rates can be focused. In illustration, a hospital food

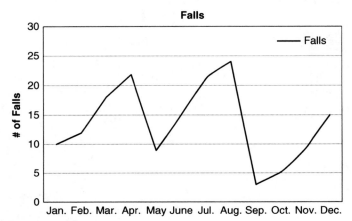

FIGURE 9.3   Sample Run Chart

service received 206 complaints about food service, which could be categorized as follows:

Complaint	Frequency
1. Food too cold	82
2. Delivered late	44
3. Tray left out of reach	26
4. Wrong order	17
5. Tasted bad	16
6. Was not delivered	10
7. Rude service	9
8. Too hot	2

Putting this information into a Pareto chart (see Figure 9.4) visualizes that 80% of the food service complaints are related to food being delivered cold. By addressing this issue, the food service staff could meet its goal of 90% satisfaction, seen as a straight line at the top of the chart at 90 on the x axis.

Control Chart

A control chart is a graphic demonstration of statistical control of a process. Statistical control refers to monitoring a process over time to prevent deterioration and facilitate improvement (Wood, 2001). Basically, a control chart is a sophisticated run chart. Data are plotted over time

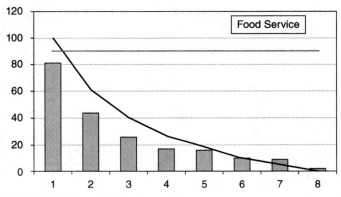

FIGURE 9.4 Sample Pareto Chart

so that patterns and trends can be easily seen. For each process (e.g., falls, infection rates, readmissions), a graph displaying the central line or average of successive samples is plotted, and "control lines" are superimposed to indicate points that are "out of control." A control chart also has three reference lines determined by historical data: a central line that represents the average, an upper line that represents the upper control limit, and a lower line that represents the lower control limit. By comparing current data to the reference lines, one can assess whether the process variation is in control (consistent) or out of control (unpredictable); for example, a control chart can be used to plot the average length of time patients spend waiting before being seen at an ambulatory clinic. Figure 9.5 presents a six-quarter (18 months) view of falls. The fall rate is in control as the mean does not extend beyond the upper (UCL) and lower control limits (LCL). The value and wide-ranging use of a control chart was articulated by Stoumbous, Reynolds, Ryan, and Woodall (2000):

> Control charts are among the most important and widely used tools in statistics. Their applications have now moved far beyond manufacturing into engineering, environmental science, biology, genetics, epidemiology, medicine, finance, and even law enforcement and athletics. (p. 992)

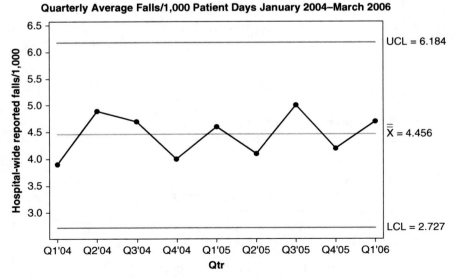

FIGURE 9.5   Sample Control Chart

Other strategies and tools for quality improvement can be found at the American Society for Quality website (asq.org/learn-about-quality/quality-tools.html), including:

- Decision-making tools
- Process-analysis tools
- Idea-creation tools
- Project-planning and implementation tools

CONCLUSION

To carry out a quality-improvement project requires thought and attention to detail. Significant time needs to be devoted to the specific aims and expected measurable outcomes of the project. Without such attention to detail, the project will lack focus. Clancy (2012) discussed seven mainstays of a safer health care system in a recent column published on the agency's website. Attention to any of these can form the basis of a quality-improvement project as follows:

- Report near misses and other adverse events.
- Take corrective-action steps to prevent future incidents from happening again.
- Communicate errors to patients.
- Apologize and waive hospital and physicians' fees when an error or other mishap occurs.
- Bridge systemic gaps that contribute to adverse events.
- Collect data and measure performance to determine whether improvements have been made.
- Educate and train staff on patient safety.

REFLECTIVE EXERCISES

1. Think about a clinical problem you want to improve; for example, length of stay, readmission rates, fall rates, operating room start times, nurse retention, staffing mix.
   - Who will be on your team?
   - What data will you need to implement your project?
   - Where can that data be found?
   - How will you collect the data that you need?
   - How will you display the data?
   - How will you disseminate the data?

2. Attend a quality-improvement meeting. Answer the following questions:
   - Who are the members of the committee?
   - What quality-improvement method are they using?
   - What quality indicators are they discussing?
   - What information are they using to inform their discussions?
   - What are the outcomes of the discussion?
3. Review the fishbone diagram in this chapter. What strategies would you put into place to address this issue? How would you monitor and sustain your strategies?

REFERENCES

American Society for Quality. (2013). *Failure mode effects analysis (FMEA)*. Retrieved from http://asq.org/learn-about-quality/process-analysis-tools/overview/fmea.html

Clancy, C. (2012). *Revealing medical errors helps Chicago hospitals build a safer health system 2012*. July 2012. Agency for Healthcare Research and Quality, Rockville, MD. Retrieved from http://www.ahrq.gov/news/columns/navigating-the-health-care-system/071012.html

Corn, J. B. (2009). Six Sigma in health care. *Radiologic Technology, 81*(1), 92–95.

Donabedian, A. (1990). The seven pillars of quality. *Archives of Pathology and Laboratory Medicine, 114*(11), 1115–1118.

Donabedian, A. (2003). *An introduction to quality assurance in healthcare*. New York, NY: Oxford University Press.

Glanville, I., Schirm, V., & Wineman, N. M. (2000). Using evidence-based practice for managing clinical outcomes in advanced practice nursing. *Journal of Nursing Care Quality, 15*(1).

Harteloh, P. P. M. (2003). The meaning of quality in health care: A conceptual analysis. *Health Care Analysis, 11*(3), 259–267.

Health Resources and Services Administration. (2011). *Quality management toolkit*. Retrieved from http://www.hrsa.gov/quality/toolbox/index.html

Hughes, R. G. (2008). Tools and strategies for quality improvement and patient safety. In R. G. Hughes (Ed.), *Patient safety and quality: An evidence-based handbook for nurses*. Rockville, MD: Agency for Healthcare Research and Quality.

Institute for Healthcare Improvement. (2004). *Failure modes and effects analysis*. Cambridge, MA: Author. Retrieved from http://www.ihi.org/knowledge/Pages/Tools/FailureModesandEffectsAnalysisTool.aspx

Institute for Healthcare Improvement. (2011). *Failure Modes and Effects Analysis (FMEA) Tool*. Cambridge, MA: Author. Retrieved from http://www.ihi.org/knowledge/Pages/Tools/FailureModesandEffectsAnalysisTool.aspx

Johansson, A. C. (2011). Perspective: Medical education research and the institutional review board; reexamining the process. *Academic Medicine, 86*, 809–817.

Joint Commission, The. (2003). Using aggregate root cause analysis to improve patient safety. *Joint Commission Journal on Quality and Patient Safety, 29*(8), 434–439.

Langley, G., Nolan, K., Nolan, T., Norman, C., & Procost, L. (2009). *The improvement guide: A practical approach to enhancing organizational performance* (2nd ed.). San Francisco, CA: Jossey-Bass.

Lynn, J., Baily, M. A., Bottrell, M., Jennings, B., Levine, R. J., Davidoff, F., . . . James, B. (2007). The ethics of using quality improvement methods in health care. *Annals of Internal Medicine, 146,* 666–673.

Mitchell, P. (2008). Defining patient safety and quality care. In R. G. Hughes (Ed.), *Patient safety and quality: An evidence-based handbook for nurses.* Rockville, MD: Agency for Healthcare Research and Quality.

Neuhauser, D., Myhre, S., & Alemi, F. (2004). *Personal continuous quality improvement workbook* (7th ed.). Washington, DC: Academy for Healthcare Improvement. Retrieved from http://www.a4hi.org/docs/Neuhauser_personal_improvement_project_workbook.pdf

Platteborze, L., Young-McCaughan, S., King-Letzkus, I., McClinton, A., Halliday, A., & Jefferson, T. C. (2010). Performance Improvement/Research Advisory Panel: A model for determining whether a project is a performance or quality improvement activity or research. *Military Medicine, 175,* 289–291.

Reinhardt, A. C., & Ray, L. N. (2003). Differentiating quality improvement from research. *Applied Nursing Research, 16*(1), 2–8.

Shojania, K. G., McDonald, K. M., Wachter, R. M., et al. (2004). *Closing the quality gap: A critical analysis of quality improvement strategies, Volume 1—Series Overview and Methodology Technical Review 9* (Contract No. 290-02-0017 to the Stanford University–UCSF Evidence-based Practice Center) (AHRQ Publication No. 04-0051-1). Rockville, MD: Agency for Healthcare Research and Quality.

Stoumbous, Z. G., Reynolds, M. R., Jr., Ryan, T. P., & Woodall, W. H. (2000). The state of statistical process control as we proceed into the 21st century. *Journal of the American Statistical Association, 95*(451), 992–998.

Wood, M. (2001). Statistical process monitoring in the 21st century. In J. Antony & D. Preece (Eds.), *Understanding, managing & implementing quality* (pp. 103–121). London, UK: Routledge.

SUGGESTED READING

Anand, G., Ward, P. T., & Tatikonda, M. V. (2010). Role of explicit and tacit knowledge in Six Sigma projects: An empirical examination of differential project success. *Journal of Operations Management, 28*(4), 303–315.

Day, S., Dalto, J., Fox, J., & Turpin, M. (2006). Failure mode and effects analysis as a performance improvement tool in trauma. *Journal of Trauma Nursing, 13*(3), 111–117.

Harrington, L. (2007). Quality improvement, research, and the institutional review board. *Journal for Healthcare Quality, 29*(3), 4–9.

Marshall, M., Shekelle, P. G., Leatherman, S., & Brook, R. H. (2000). The public release of performance data: What do we expect to gain, a review of the evidence. *Journal of the American Medical Association, 283,* 1866–1874.

Reinhardt, A. C., & Ray, L. N. (2003). Differentiating quality improvement from research. *Applied Nursing Research, 16*(1), 2–8.

Rooney, J. J., & Vanden Heuvel, L. N. (2004). *Root cause analysis for beginners.* Available at: www.asq.org

Utilization of a Nurse-Driven Protocol to Decrease Catheter-Associated Urinary Tract Infections

DONNA BARTO

Background: Catheter-associated urinary tract infections are the most common hospital-acquired infection and can lead to patient problems, including increased length of stay, increased mortality risk, and ultimately higher hospital costs. Catheter-associated urinary tract infections (CAUTI) are responsible for 13% of the nearly 100,000 hospital-associated infection deaths occurring in the United States each year (Rothfeld & Stickley, 2010). Catheters are a medically necessary intervention in many cases. However, they are at times unnecessary and are probably left in longer than they are needed. The longer a catheter remains in place, the higher the risk of urinary tract infection becomes. Publicly reported hospital data on CAUTI will be readily available for the public to view on the web. This can impact the hospital's revenue in that consumers may select not to receive care at a hospital that has been shown to have a higher incidence of catheter-associated urinary tract infections.

The current procedure for removing a urinary catheter at a community hospital is to have a physician's order to remove it. Many times the physician forgets that the urinary catheter is in place, and the catheter is left in longer than necessary. One way to overcome this barrier is to authorize the nurse to remove the catheter based on a set of criteria. Nurses would not need a physician order, therefore eliminating another step in the catheter-removal process and not leaving the catheter in longer than necessary.

Purpose: The purpose of this project was to:

- Develop a nurse-driven protocol that allows nurses to remove urinary catheters without a physician's order
- Monitor the use of the protocol over a 5-month period

Method: This was a quality-improvement study using a PDCA cycle. The protocol was designed by a multidisciplinary group after the review of the literature (*Plan*). Numerous revisions to the protocol were carried out based on input from managers, advanced practice nurses, staff nurses, physicians, and various hospital practice committees. After the protocol was approved, training tools for educational sessions were developed by four advanced practice nurses. Education consisted of a variety of formats, including online learning, information sheets posted in the units, and face-to-face learning (*Do*). Compliance in using the protocol was monitored during multidisciplinary rounds, which were conducted daily. Data were collected on the prevalence of urinary catheters as well as the rate of catheter-associated urinary tract infections prior to the implementation of the nurse-driven protocol. Data were also collected on the rate of catheter-associated urinary tract infections for 5 months after the implementation of the nurse-driven protocol. The data-analysis method consisted of an independent-sample, two-tailed *t*-test. This study compared one sample (preprotocol) to another sample (postprotocol) to see whether there is a decrease in the number of urinary catheters used in the intensive care unit and the rate of hospital-wide catheter-associated urinary tract infections postintervention (*Check*).

Results: Data analysis revealed that the mean infection rate for the preprotocol group ($N = 6,463$) was 1.231; the mean rate for the postprotocol group ($N = 5,167$) was 0.348. This decrease in infection rate in the postintervention group is calculated to have a 95% confidence interval and is statistically significant with a *p* value of less than 0.0001. In looking at the intensive care unit's catheter utilization ratio, the utilization ratio of catheters decreased. The power of this study was calculated to be less than 0.0001. Given the high power of the study, as well as a 95% confidence interval, the project does demonstrate that a nurse-driven protocol allowing nurses to remove urinary catheters without a physician order does decrease the urinary catheter days as well as the rate of urinary tract infections in a community hospital. These measures will continue to be monitored and reported back to staff to sustain these lower rates (*Act*).

Conclusions: By allowing nurses to carry out the process of removing urinary catheters without a physician's order, the hospital gains through future increases in value-based purchasing incentives as well as not being penalized financially for urinary tract infections. However, the biggest advantage lies with the improvement in patient care in terms of decreased morbidity, mortality, pain, and suffering associated with a catheter-associated urinary tract infection.

REFERENCE

Rothfeld, A., & Stickley, A. (2010). A program to limit urinary catheter use at an acute care hospital. *American Journal of Infection Control, 38*, 568–571.

10

Program Evaluation

OBJECTIVES

At the end of the chapter, you will be able to:
- Define program evaluation
- Differentiate among goal-based, process, outcome, formative, and summative evaluations
- Write evaluation goals
- Develop an evaluation plan

KEY CONCEPTS

Most evaluations fall into one of five categories:

- Formative evaluation structured to provide information for immediate project improvement.

- Summative evaluation conducted for the purpose of accountability, which requires determining the overall effectiveness or merit and worth of an evaluation object.

- Outcome evaluation to measure whether or not the project achieved its intended outcome.

- Goal-based evaluation to determine the extent to which programs are meeting predetermined goals or objectives.

- Process-based evaluation focused on a complete understanding about how a program works.

Every evaluation is different as it is guided by the specific purpose of the evaluation, the evaluation questions asked, and the developmental stage of the program.

A program evaluation is the process of collecting, analyzing, and using data to measure the impact or outcomes of a program using valid and reliable methods to examine the process or outcomes of an organization

(Grinnell & Unrau, 2008, p. 553). According to Patton (2008), program evaluation is the "systematic collection of information about the activities, characteristics, and results of programs to make judgments about the program" (p. 39), whereas Rossi (2004) believes that evaluation is a method of social research designed to answer questions of policy. Typically, evaluation involves assessment of one of the following: (a) program need, (b) program plan, (c) program performance, (d) program impact, or (e) program effectiveness (Rossi, Lipsey, & Freeman, 2004). The motivation involved in conducting a program evaluation is to show the success and benefits of a particular approach and to determine a program's quality. The purpose of an evaluation can be for accountability or program development (Centers for Disease Control and Prevention, 2011; Patton, 2008).

A carefully planned and conducted program evaluation can:

1. Answer such questions as: Is the program having its intended effect? How can it be improved? Are there better and more cost-effective options to run the program?
2. Identify program strengths and weaknesses to improve or strengthen the program.
3. Produce data or verify results that can be used to expand the program.
4. Produce valid comparisons among programs to decide which should be retained in the face of pending budget cuts.
5. Describe effective programs for duplication elsewhere.

GUIDING PRINCIPLES OF EVALUATION

The American Association of Evaluation (2013) has developed a set of guidelines to design and conduct evaluation activities (www.eval.org/GPTraining/GP%20Training%20Final/gp.principles.pdf). These indicate that the evaluation should:

- Address both the strengths and weaknesses of the program
- Demonstrate cultural competence in the selection of evaluation strategies
- Report any real or potential conflicts of interest regarding the evaluation

- Seek a comprehensive understanding of the contextual elements of the evaluation
- Abide by current professional ethics standards and regulations regarding confidentiality, informed consent, and protection of human subjects
- Seek to maximize the benefits and reduce any harm that might occur from an evaluation

Evaluators should possess the appropriate knowledge and skill to conduct an evaluation. These include an understanding of research methods and analysis, the ability to think critically and make judgments based on findings, and the capacity to move beyond superficial information to understand fully how a program operates.

Evaluation should be practical and feasible and conducted within the parameters of resources, time, and political context. Evaluation findings should be used to make decisions about program implementation and to improve program effectiveness. In this way, program evaluation is different from research in that a research study is conducted to test a hypothesis or generate meaning, whereas a program evaluation is conducted to improve practice (MacDonald et al., 2001). Table 10.1 displays some of the principles that distinguish research and program evaluation.

TABLE 10.1 Research Versus Program Evaluation

	Research	Program Evaluation
Purpose	Test hypothesis or generate meaning	Greater understanding
Guiding questions	Facts (descriptions, associations, effects)	Value (merit, worth, significance)
	Meaning	
Strengths	Internal validity (accuracy, precision)	Context Utility
	External validity (generalizability)	
Use	Disseminate to interested audiences	Feedback to stakeholders

Adapted from MacDonald et al. (2001).

TYPES OF EVALUATION

Formative Evaluation

Formative evaluation is structured to provide information for project improvement. Emphasis is on findings that are timely, concrete, and immediately useful (Rossiet al., 2004). The purpose of a formative evaluation is to better *form* the program to meet its expected outcomes. A formative evaluation allows consideration and review of program planning efforts while in the early stages of implementation, rather than waiting until the program has been fully developed and completed. Also known as a usability study, a formative evaluation can uncover unintended consequences. For example, Landau (2001) provides two examples of unintended results of a program identified during a formative evaluation: one negative and one positive. First, she explains that during the early days of antidrug films, young people learned new ways of drug use by watching movies that illustrated behavior that was intended to discourage drug use. On a more positive note, she described that while television stations, under the Americans with Disabilities Act, provide closed-captioned programming to make broadcasts accessible to people who are hearing impaired or deaf, these captions are also used by those who are just learning to read or who are learning a second language.

Formative evaluation is a relatively new concept as applied to health care programs and may not be appropriate for evaluating all health care programs. Stetler et al. (2006), for example, explain that in a randomized controlled trial, researchers do not typically change or modify the experimental arm once it has been approved; however, changes in a quality-improvement project as it is being conducted may be important in obtaining the right data essential to improving processes.

Formative evaluation differs from the other types of evaluation as it is ongoing and involves an informed judgment on the part of the evaluator as to whether or not the program is likely to meet its intended goals (Beyer, 1995). Considerations in planning a formative evaluation include:

- Plan the evaluation before development of the program is completed
- Conduct the formative evaluation at several times during the program development phase
- Focus on the collection of information that will be of immediate use when planning and developing the program
- Use the results of each evaluation to revise or modify the program (Beyer, 1995)

Summative Evaluation

Summative evaluation is a summary. It is retrospective in nature in contrast to the prospective view needed for a formative evaluation. Summative evaluation determines whether an intervention, service, or program is working. Summative evaluation takes place most often at the end of a project. As such, summative evaluation is referred to as ex-post (after the event) evaluation, and is linked to accountability. For example, a summative evaluation is about the decreased rates and sustainability of smoking following a smoking-cessation program, rather than a description of how many attended the program. Some reasons to undertake a summative evaluation include (Evaluation Toolbox, 2010):

- As a means to determine whether a project or program has met its goals/objectives/outcomes
- To determine the impact of a program
- To compare the impact of different projects and make decisions on future spending allocation
- To develop a better understanding of the process of change, and finding out what works, what doesn't work, and why; this provides the knowledge to improve future projects and implementation
- To determine whether a program is still operating as it was originally intended.

Goal-Based Evaluation

Goal-based evaluations determine the extent to which programs are meeting predetermined goals or objectives. Goals-based evaluation does not question whether the selected goals are legitimate; it determines whether or not the goal, as stated, has been met (Evaluation Toolbox, 2010). A goal-based evaluation can be either formative or summative.

A goal is a statement that can be used to ascertain an organization's progress. Goals can be related to money, equipment, facilities, staffing, timelines, or other resources. Setting goals provides a purpose and a focus to actions. A goal is a global statement of what is to be accomplished and it may have subordinate, more focused goals attached to it. Goals should be written in a positive manner and, using the future tense, provide a time frame for accomplishment and be clear in what is intended. The 3 Ps of good goals are that they are positive, precise, and performance oriented.

Examples of program goals are:

- At the end of 1 year, $500,000 for program operations will have been awarded
- Six months following completion of a smoking-cessation program, 50% of participants will have stopped smoking
- Emergency department wait times will have decreased to 15 minutes or less by the end of the year

Goal-based evaluation does not question whether the goals are valid or whether appropriate measures of effectiveness are being assessed. A goal-based evaluation just determines whether or not the goals are being met.

Process Evaluation

Process, or implementation, evaluations are focused on a complete understanding of how a program works. They are useful for replication of the program in other settings and for monitoring of a program's effectiveness. Process evaluations are the most commonly used method of evaluation as they can be used as a stand-alone form of assessment or in combination with an outcome evaluation. A process evaluation answers the question: Does the program deliver its intended objectives to the target population? Basically, a process evaluation assesses the fidelity and effectiveness of a program's implementation (Rossi, Lipsey, & Freeman, 2004). According to Rossi et al. (2004):

> [A process evaluation] might examine how consistently services actually delivered are consistent with the goals of the program, whether services are delivered to appropriate recipients, how will service delivery be organized, the effectiveness of program management, the use of program resources, and other such matters. (p. 57)

Process evaluation focuses on the internal operations of a program to determine its strengths and weaknesses and areas needing improvement. A process evaluation can map an actual operation, for example, the discharge process or the experiences of families in the intensive care unit. It is a search for patterns, trends, successes, and failures (Patton, 2008). For example, Plochg, Delnoij, van der Kruk, Janmaat, and Klazinga (2005) evaluated the process of an intermediate care model between a university hospital and a residential home using t-tests and a chi-squared test to assess significance. Semistructured interviews were conducted with 21 staff members representing all disciplines. Results indicated that despite high expectations, a heterogeneous, more complex than expected patient population; an unqualified staff; and cultural differences among collaborating partners impeded implementation. The evaluators concluded that setting up a discharge model of intermediate care between a university hospital and a residential home is less straightforward than was originally perceived.

Outcomes-Based Evaluation

Outcome, or impact evaluation, determines whether or not the project has achieved its intended outcome. It involves developing and analyzing data to assess program impact and is a formal determination of effectiveness. For example, the impact of a statewide media campaign for youth suicide prevention was analyzed through call volumes to a national hotline to determine whether the advertisements have raised awareness of the hotline. Multilevel model estimates suggested that the campaign significantly and substantially increased calls to the hotline (Jenner, Jenner, Matthews-Sterling, Butts, & Evans Williams, 2010).

In an outcome evaluation, efforts focus on a single program. Such analysis cannot be attempted without the baseline data for comparison. For example, in a heart failure program, two outcomes measures were chosen, and they were monitored before and after the implementation of the program. The measures were:

1. The patient discharged with a diagnosis of heart failure will see a primary care provider within 2 weeks of discharge
2. Patients discharged with a diagnosis of heart failure will not be readmitted for the same diagnosis within a 90-day period

Program success was defined as whether, or to what extent, these two goals were met. Other approaches to basic outcome evaluation might include comparisons within a program; for example, what are the characteristics of those who were not followed up by a primary care provider within a 2-week period or who were readmitted with the same diagnosis within 90 days of discharge? This extension of the outcome evaluation can predict those at high risk at the outset of the program and follow-up efforts can be focused.

The value of an outcome evaluation lies in its ability to provide information program performance using before-and-after comparisons. It allows the evaluator to answer the question: "Did the program make a difference?" Although it doesn't explain what would happen if the program was not implemented, it provides information regarding program impact on preselected criteria. The United Way of America (2013; www.unitedway.org/outcomes) provides an excellent overview of outcomes-based evaluation, including introduction to outcomes measurement, a program outcome model, reasons to measure outcomes, and use of program outcome findings.

DEVELOPING AN EVALUATION PLAN

An evaluation plan is a document that outlines the way in which the evaluation will be conducted. The Centers for Disease Control and Prevention (2011) has developed a framework for writing an evaluation plan that involves engaging stakeholders, describing the program, focusing the evaluation design, gathering credible evidence, justifying conclusions, and disseminating results to ensure use of the findings.

The first step in any program evaluation is to determine the goals of the evaluation and write the questions that the evaluation is designed to answer; in other words, what are you going to evaluate? This question will determine the type of evaluation to be conducted. For example, if the intent of the evaluation is to determine how a program works, then a process evaluation is appropriate. A selective focus for the evaluation is usually necessary because an evaluation of an entire program (a formative evaluation) is costly and time intensive; for example, the evaluation may address teaching style, patient satisfaction, or more complex behavioral changes related to a specific intervention. Whatever the focus of the evaluation, it is necessary to write goals and questions that guide the process.

The SMART model provides a framework for developing evaluation goals. Goals should be specific, measurable, achievable, results-focused, and timely. In other words, *SMART*. To be specific, goals should be precise and simple, and should clearly define what will be accomplished. They should be jargon free and have only one meaning. To be measurable, audit criteria should be quantifiable so that tangible evidence of accomplishments is obtained. Achievable goals are those that are possible and practical. Goals should measure results or outcomes, rather than activities. Timely audit criteria are those that have a specified time frame for accomplishment such as daily, on admission, quarterly, or annually. Goals should be linked to a time frame (Holly, Rittenmeyer, & Weeks, in press). Evaluation questions should be specific to the intent of the evaluation. See Table 10.2 for examples on how to focus an evaluation question. Other considerations when writing the evaluation plan are:

- What information is needed to answer the evaluation questions
- Where the information will be found
- The methods for collecting information

TABLE 10.2   Focusing Evaluation Questions

Type of Evaluation	Focus
Outcome/impact evaluation	What do people do differently as a result of the program?
	What are the strengths and weaknesses of the program?
	Did the program reach its intended audience?
Process evaluation	What methods were used to deliver the program?
	Were resources adequate to meet program goals?
Goal-based evaluation	Were intended goals met?
	Do goals have to be refined?
Formative evaluation	Who benefited from the program?
	What lessons can be learned from this initiative?
	Is the program sustainable?

TABLE 10.3   Characteristics of Commonly Used Methods of Data Collection for Program Evaluation

Method	Characteristics
Questionnaire	Nonthreatening
	Anonymous
	Inexpensive
	Information can be obtained from a large sample
Interviews/focus groups	Time-consuming
	Provides in-depth information about processes, procedures, and conditions
Document review	Uses patient care records, meeting minutes, financial records, and status reports to determine how a program operates
Observation	Time-consuming
	Examination of a program in operation

To answer the evaluation questions, the right data need to be collected. Table 10.3 provides an overview of the commonly used evaluation data-collection methods. It is useful to develop a plan for the collection of data that details the information needed and its source for each of the evaluation questions (see Table 10.4). Both quantitative and qualitative data are collected for a program evaluation. The use of both types of data, in combination, provides both a measure of change and important contextual information. Some considerations when collecting data for evaluation include:

TABLE 10.4 Data-Collection Plan

Evaluation Question	Outcome/ Goal or Indicator	Information Needed	Data Source	Method of Data Collection	Frequency of Data Collection	Responsible Party
What do you want to know?	How will you know it?	What do you need to know?	Where can you find these data?	How will you collect the data you need?	How often will you collect the needed data?	Who will be in charge of making sure the data are collected and analyzed?
How well is the suicide hotline program working?	Call volume will increase by 20% in 3 months	Number of calls before and after implementation of a media campaign for prevention of suicide	Electronic call registry	Retro– spective review of call registry	Aggregated weekly	Program director

Adapted from CDC (2011); Jenner (2010).

(a) Both qualitative and quantitative data are collected so that all aspects of the program can be understood, and (b) the entire program needs to be evaluated—a snapshot is not adequate (Evaluation Toolbox, 2010).

- Delineate the time frame for collecting information, that is, when will the evaluation period start and when will it end? This time frame is the period during which you will collect data to answer the question; for example, 3 months, 6 months, 1 year.
- How will the information be analyzed? Analyzing quantitative and qualitative data collected should follow the accepted methods for the type of data collected; for example, interview or focus data should be analyzed using content analysis. When analyzing data for a program evaluation, the analysis is focused on the purpose and goals of the evaluation. For example, if the intent of the evaluation was to identify strengths and weaknesses, data should be organized by results related to strengths and weaknesses of the program (Grinnell & Unrae, 2008).
- Who will get the evaluation report?

THE EVALUATION REPORT

Evaluation reports begin with an executive summary. An executive summary is a brief description of the main findings of the evaluation. It is an extended abstract that describes the important points and findings of the evaluation and includes a clear description of the program, service, or intervention being evaluated; a statement of the purpose of the evaluation; and a brief description of methods used for data collection and analysis. The major findings and conclusions linked to the evaluation goals should also be included in the executive summary. Although there is not a page requirement for an executive summary, a good summary is at least two single-spaced pages.

The remainder of the report provides extended detail regarding each of the sections of the executive summary, including:

1. The purpose of the report and the type of evaluation that was conducted. The type of evaluation conducted should be explained in some detail so that the reader understands the process used.

2. Background and history about the program, service, or intervention that was evaluated are given.

3. A description of goals or the questions being answered by the evaluation, that is, what questions were answered by the evaluation, are listed.

4. A methods section is supplied that describes the information collected, including any tools used to collect the information and how the data were analyzed.

5. Interpretations and conclusions, which should be as transparent as possible, are described. An interpretation involves putting collected data into the context of the program or service and determining whether the goals were met or the outcomes were accomplished. It is important in developing this section to fully explain any results indicating that the program or service did not have its intended effect, as well as a description of outcomes identified as a part of the evaluation that were not expected. Unanticipated outcomes or lack of meeting predetermined goals can indicate that the program suppositions used to develop the program were wrong. They can also be an indication that there was a flaw in the program design. It is, therefore, important to fully describe and interpret any negative or unexpected outcomes and identify what may have gone wrong. This will help improve the program (Grinnell & Unrae, 2008). For example, if a program relied heavily on printed handout material written in English in a program of largely non-English speakers, the program will probably not meet its goals.

6. Recommendations, which should reflect the questions asked as a part of the evaluation, are supplied and the findings for each question are explained. Recommendations provided should enable the program staff to improve the program.

USING EVALUATION RESULTS

The ultimate purpose of program evaluation is to use the information generated to improve programs. The results of an evaluation can improve organizational management and planning, assist in decision making, and indicate where improvement is needed. Patton (2002) has noted that the use of evaluation findings does not just happen; the process must be facilitated. Some strategies to facilitate the use of findings include: (a) Engage stakeholders early in the preparation for the evaluation and design the evaluation to achieve intended uses by stakeholders; (b) prepare stakeholders for eventual use by rehearsing how different conclusions could affect outcomes; (c) provide continuous feedback to stakeholders as the evaluation progresses, particularly those that might affect the use of findings; (d) schedule follow-up meetings with intended users to facilitate the transfer of evaluation findings into strategic decision making; and (e) establish a monitoring mechanism to determine how well evaluation findings and recommendations are used (MacDonald et al., 2001).

CONCLUSION

A program evaluation is about continually improving a program or service. Although it is important to demonstrate how successful the program was, it is equally important to understand why some aspects of the program did not work as well as intended. "Evaluation is not about finding out about everything, but about *finding the things that matter*" (Evaluation Toolbox, 2010, p. 1).

REFLECTIVE EXERCISES

1. Discuss how the guiding principles inform the ethical practice of evaluation.
2. Read the following article about a program evaluation. Determine how the goals were defined, how they were measured, and whether or not the program was successful.
   Larrabee, J. H., Boldreghini, S., Elder-Sorrells, K., Turner, Z. M., Wender, R. G., Hart, J. M., & Lenzi, P. S. (2001). Evaluation of documentation before and after implementation of a nursing information system in an acute care hospital. *Computers in Nursing, 19*(2), 56–65.
3. Find a newspaper account of an evaluation that was completed. Are the findings of the evaluation clear? See whether you can find the original evaluation report on the Internet. How close is the report to the newspaper account?

REFERENCES

American Association of Evaluation. (2013). *Guidelines for the design and conduct of evaluation activities*. Retrieved February 10, 2013, from http://www.eval. org/GPTraining/GP%20Training%20Final/gp.principles.pdf

Beyer, B. (1995). *How to conduct a formative evaluation*. Washington, DC: Association for the Supervision of Curriculum Development. Retrieved from http://isites.harvard.edu/fs/docs/icb.topic541040.files/A_beyer1995 pp1-36_44-57_66-70_78-81.pdf

Centers for Disease Control and Prevention. (2011). *Developing an effective evaluation plan*. Atlanta, GA: Centers for Disease Control and Prevention, National Center for Chronic Disease Prevention and Health Promotion, Office on Smoking and Health; Division of Nutrition, Physical Activity, and Obesity. Retrieved from http://www.cdc.gov/obesity/downloads/CDC-Evaluation-Workbook-508.pdf

Evaluation Toolbox. (2010). Retrieved from http://www.evaluationtoolbox. net.au/index.php?option=com_content&view=article&id=15&Itemid=19

Grinnell, R., & Unrae, Y. (2008). *Social work research and evaluation* (8th ed.). New York, NY: Oxford University Press.

Holly, C., Rittenmeyer, L., & Weeks, S. (in press). *Orthopedic Nursing*.

Jenner, E., Jenner, L. W., Matthews-Sterling, M., Butts, J., & Evans Williams, T. (2010). Awareness effects of a youth suicide prevention media campaign in Louisiana. *Suicide and Life-Threatening Behavior, 40*(4), 394–406.

Landau, V. (2001). *Developing a project management plan instructor's notes*. Retrieved March 10, 2013, from www.roundworldmedia.com/cvc/module10/notes10.html

MacDonald, G., Starr, G., Schooley, M., Yee, S. L., Klimowski, K., & Turner, K. (2001). *Introduction to program evaluation for comprehensive tobacco control programs*. Atlanta, GA: Centers for Disease Control and Prevention. Retrieved from http://www.cdc.gov/tobacco/tobacco_control_programs/surveillance_evaluation/evaluation_manual/pdfs/evaluation.pdf

Patton, M. Q. (2002). *Utilization-Focused Evaluation (U-FE) checklist*. Retrieved from http://www.mymande.org/sites/default/files/ufe.pdf

Patton, M. Q. (2008). *Utilization-Focused Evaluation* (4th ed.). Thousand Oaks, CA: Sage.

Plochg, T., Delnoij, D., van der Kruk, T., Janmaat, T., & Klazinga, N. (2005). Intermediate care: For better or worse? Process evaluation of an intermediate care model between a university hospital and a residential home. *BMC Health Service Research, 5,* 38.

Rossi, P., Lipsey, M., & Freeman, H. (2004). *Evaluation. A systematic approach* (7th ed.). Thousand Oaks, CA: Sage.

Stetler, C. B., Legro, M. W., Wallace, C. M., Bowman, C., Guihan, M., Hagedorn, H., Kimmel, B., . . . Smith, J. L. (2006). The role of formative evaluation in implementation research and the QUERI experience. *Journal of General Internal Medicine, 21,* S1–S8.

United Way of America. (2013). Retrieved January 25, 2012, from http://www.unitedway.org/outcomes

SUGGESTED READING

Lin, Y. R., Shiah, I. S., Chang, Y. C., Lai, T. J., Wang, K. Y., & Chou, K. R. (2004). Evaluation of an assertiveness training program on nursing and medical students' assertiveness, self-esteem, and interpersonal communication satisfaction. *Nurse Educator Today, 24*(8), 656–665.

Nelson, A., Matz, M., Chen, F., Siddharthan, K., Lloyd, J., & Fragala, G. (2006). Development and evaluation of a multifaceted ergonomics program to prevent injuries associated with patient handling tasks. *International Journal of Nursing Studies, 43*(6), 717–733.

Ross, A., & Crumpler, J. (2007). The impact of an evidence-based practice education program on the role of oral care in the prevention of ventilator-associated pneumonia. *Intensive & Critical Care Nursing, 23*(3), 132–136.

Summative Evaluation of Patient Satisfaction Strategies in an Urban Emergency Department

AHMAD SINGER

Background: Externally conducted surveys of patient satisfaction are the norm in hospitals today and are linked to hospital reimbursement. This initiative provides an incentive to improve patient care and develop processes to improve the patient experience. A significant decrease in patient satisfaction scores was observed over a two-quarter period in a large urban emergency department. This decrease in scores occurred after a lengthy process to address low patient satisfaction scores the previous year. A protocol was developed for all staff to follow, which initially resulted in a significant increase in scores. The decrease in scores prompted an evaluation as to why this was occurring.

Aim: The purpose of this study was to conduct an evaluation of the measures used initially that were instrumental in increasing patient satisfaction-related scores and to determine whether those measures are still the best strategies to use and to suggest alternative strategies as appropriate. An additional aim was to determine the emergency department staff's accountability for the protocol. A proxy definition of patient satisfaction was used in this project that included these nurse-sensitive indicators: (a) courtesy, (b) taking time to listen, and (c) being informative regarding treatment.

Method: Summative evaluation was an ex-post (after the event) evaluation associated with accountability. Direct and random observations of staff were conducted to determine whether the protocol developed 1 year prior to increase patient satisfaction scores was still being followed. These observations were documented on a checklist designed for specific areas within the emergency department, such as triage, urgent care, main emergency department, and waiting room. The protocol developed as a part of the initial effort to increase scores was used as the checklist for this observation. The observation was conducted at random times and on random days. The day of the observation was randomly selected from a bag containing all of the days of the week. In turn, the time of observation was selected randomly from another bag containing 1-hour time frames for observation. The staff observed were selected from among those on duty during the selected time and day using the same method. All observed staff were seen in interaction with patients while completing a full range of patient care activities in all of the emergency department areas.

Findings: The results of the direct observations showed variations in the adoption of the protocol by the majority of staff observed. These findings supported that the significant drop in the proxy patient satisfaction scores during the fourth quarter could have contributed to the variations and inconsistencies in using the protocol.

Conclusion: A consistent standard work guideline is necessary in order to improve the perception of care by the patients and their families. It was obvious during this evaluation that the established protocol was not being followed. The emergency department performance improvement committee recommended that the work protocol be further refined and introduced to new staff through hiring and orientation, and that continuing staff be held accountable for the tenets of the protocol through yearly evaluation.

A

Selected Resources for Scholarly Inquiry in Advanced Practice

ACTION RESEARCH

Herr, K., & Anderson, G. (2005). *The action research dissertation: A guide for students and faculty*. Thousand Oaks, CA: Sage.

Stringer, E. (2013). *Action research* (4th ed.). Thousand Oaks, CA: Sage.

CASE STUDY

Yin, R. (2009). *Case study research: Design and methods*. Thousand Oaks, CA: Sage.

CLINICAL INTERVENTION RESEARCH

Melnyk, B., & Morrison-Beedy, D. (2012). *Intervention research: Designing, conducting, analyzing, and funding*. New York, NY: Springer Publishing Company.

INTEGRATIVE REVIEW

Garrard, J. (2011). *Health science literature review made easy: The matrix method*. Sudbury, MA: Jones & Bartlett.

PROGRAM EVALUATION

Hickey, J. V., & Brosnan, C. A. (2012). *Evaluation of health care quality in advanced practice nursing.* New York, NY: Springer Publishing Company.
Rossi, P., Lipsey, M., & Freeman, H. (2003). *Evaluation: A systematic approach* (7th ed.). Thousand Oaks, CA: Sage.

QUALITATIVE DESCRIPTIVE

Saldana, J. (2013). *The coding manual for qualitative researchers.* Thousand Oaks, CA: Sage.
Sandelowski, M., & Barroso, J. (2007). *Handbook for synthesizing qualitative research.* New York, NY: Springer Publishing Company.

QUALITY IMPROVEMENT

McLaughlin, C., & Kaluzny, A. (2005). *Continuous quality improvement in health care: Theory, implementations, and applications* (3rd ed.). Sudbury, MA: Jones & Bartlett.
Tague, N. (2005). *The quality improvement toolkit.* Wisconsin, MA: ASQ.

SUGGESTED READING

Norris, A., Aroian, K., Warren, S., & Wirth, J. (2012). Interactive performance and focus groups with adolescents: The power of play. *Research in Nursing & Health, 35*(6), 671–679.
Polit, D. F., & Chaboyer, W. (2012). Statistical process control in nursing research. *Research in Nursing & Health, 35*(1), 82–93. doi: 10.1002/nur.20467

SYSTEMATIC REVIEW

Cumming, G. (2012). *Understanding the statistics: Effect size, confidence intervals and meta-analysis.* New York, NY: Routledge, Francis and Taylor Group.
Holly, C., Salmond, S., & Saimbert, M. (2012). *Comprehensive systematic review for advanced nursing practice.* New York, NY: Springer Publishing Company.
Sandelowski, M., & Barroso, J. (2007). *Handbook for synthesizing qualitative research.* New York, NY: Springer Publishing Company.

B

Selected Resources for Human Subject Protection

ELEMENTS OF A CONSENT FORM

www.coloradocollege.edu/other/irb/consent

HUMAN SUBJECT PROTECTION TRAINING

National Institutes of Health (NIH)
  phrp.nihtraining.com/users/login.php

Collaborative Institutional Training Initiative (CITI)
  www.citiprogram.org/default.asp?language=english

OFFICE OF HUMAN SUBJECT PROTECTION

www.hhs.gov/ohrp

PRINCIPLES OF ETHICAL RESEARCH

www.apa.org/monitor/jan03/principles.aspx

SUGGESTED READING

Davis, A., Hull, S. C., Grady, C., Wilfond, B. S., & Henderson, G. E. (2002). The invisible hand in clinical research: The study coordinator's critical role in human subjects protection. *Journal of Law, Medicine & Ethics, 30*, 411–419.

Lynn, J. (2004). When does quality improvement count as research? Human subject protection and theories of knowledge. *Quality and Safety in Health Care, 13*, 67–70. doi:10.1136/qshc.2002.002436

TIPS FOR WRITING AN INSTITUTIONAL REVIEW BOARD APPLICATION

mindlesseating.org/pdf/IRB_Applications.doc

Selected How-To Sources for Clinical Studies

HOW TO ANALYZE DATA
Quantitative Data

Confidence Intervals

www.health.ny.gov/diseases/chronic/confint.htm

www.nottingham.ac.uk/nursing/sonet/rlos/ebp/confidence_intervals/index.html

Statistics Calculator

www.graphpad.com/quickcalcs/index.cfm

Statistical Tests

statisticalhelp.com

learningstore.uwex.edu/assets/pdfs/G3658-12.PDF

www.insites.org/CLIP_v1_site/downloads/PDFs/TipsAnalz QualData.5D.8-07.pdf

HOW TO CHOOSE THE RIGHT RESEARCH DESIGN

libguides.usc.edu/content.php?pid=83009&sid=818072

hsl.lib.umn.edu/biomed/help/understanding-research-study-designs

www.vadscorner.com/internet7.html

HOW TO EVALUATE EVIDENCE

www.hsl.unc.edu/Services/Tutorials/EBM/Evidence.htm

HOW TO KNOW YOU ARE ON THE RIGHT TRACK

Examples of Clinical Projects

doctorsofnursingpractice.org/studentprojects.php

HOW TO SEARCH THE LITERATURE

www.hsl.unc.edu/Services/Tutorials/EBM/Question.htm

HOW TO WRITE A CAPSTONE/RESEARCH PROPOSAL

researchproposalguide.com

www.design.umn.edu/current_students/info/documents/AGuideto
WritingaCapstoneProposal-CDES.pdf

www.apastyle.org/learn/tutorials/basics-tutorial.aspx

sn.umdnj.edu/academics/dnp/files/ProposalTemplate.doc

HOW TO WRITE A CLINICAL/RESEARCH QUESTION

www.hsl.unc.edu/Services/Tutorials/EBM/Question.htm

www.cebm.utoronto.ca/practise/formulate

writingcenter.gmu.edu/?p=307

HOW TO WRITE A LITERATURE REVIEW

library.usm.maine.edu/tutorials/esp/module3/21_write.htm

HOW TO WRITE THE FINAL REPORT

writingcenter.unc.edu/handouts/dissertations

INDEX